The Manhattan Diaries Series

Eat Like an A-Lister
Manhattan's Ultimate Nutrition Guide

Manhattan Vitality
Just Like That

The Manhattan Diaries Series

Manhattan Allure ~ Just Like That

Manhattan Vitality ~ Just Like That

Manhattan Lifestyle ~ Just Like That

Manhattan Ambition ~ Just Like That

The Manhattan Diaries Series

Eat Like an A-Lister
Manhattan's Ultimate Nutrition Guide

Manhattan Vitality
Just Like That

CANDICE MALONE

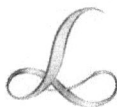

L

Urban Chronicles Publishing House
an imprint of The Ridge Publishing Group
Coeur d'Alene, Idaho, U.S.A.

DISCLAIMER: The ideas, concepts, and opinions expressed in The Manhattan Diaries Series (hereinafter referred to as "Series") are intended to help readers make thoughtful and informed decisions about their lifestyle. This Series is sold with the understanding that author and publisher are not rendering medical advice of any kind, nor is this Series intended to replace the medical advice, nor to diagnose, prescribe, or treat any disease, condition, illness, or injury. It should not be used as a substitute for treatment by or the advice of a professional healthcare provider. It is recommended that before beginning any diet or exercise program, including any aspect of the Series, you receive full medical clearance from a licensed healthcare provider. Although the author and publisher have endeavored to ensure that the information provided in the Series is complete and accurate, the author and publisher claim no responsibility to any person or entity for any liability, loss, or damage caused or alleged to be caused directly or indirectly as a result of the use, application, or interpretation of the material in this Series, or any errors or omissions in the Series.

CREDIT: This book was written with limited assistance of ChatGPT, an AI language model developed by OpenAI. The collaboration provided unique insights and support in crafting content. The book cover was created using Midjourney tools and Adobe Photoshop, ensuring a visually captivating design.

Library of Congress Control Number: 2024923937

Eat Like an A-Lister: Manhattan's Ultimate Nutrition Guide by Candice Malone

ISBN: 978-1-956905-47-2 (e-book)
ISBN: 978-1-956905-46-5 (Softcover)

1. Health & Fitness / Nutrition. 2. Self-Help / Personal Growth / Happiness. 3. Cooking / Regional & Ethnic / American / Middle Atlantic States. 4. Lifestyle & Personal Style Guides. 5. Travel / United States / Northeast / Middle Atlantic / New York. I. Title. II. Series.

First Edition: October 2024

Printed in the United States of America

Contents

The Manhattan Diaries Series

DARE TO REIMAGINE YOURSELF . . .

21 Steps to Reinvent and Discover a Side of You Manhattan's Never Seen

The Manhattan Diaries Series presents:

Manhattan Allure—Just Like That mini-series (books 1–5)

Manhattan Vitality—Just Like That mini-series (books 6–10)

Manhattan Lifestyle—Just Like That mini-series (books 11–16)

Manhattan Ambition—Just Like That mini-series (books 17–21)

Meet the Author
https://www.LAMoeszinger.com

Meet the Publisher, Urban Chronicles Publishing House
https://www.NewYouniversityChronicles.com

Step into the whirlwind world of New York's glitzy underbelly, where the scintillating secrets and laugh-out-loud confessions of a metropolitan woman are laid bare by someone truly in the know. Through essays pulled from her chic "Manhattanite's Survival Guide—Success in the City," L invites us on an unforgettable strut from her glamorous youth, through her middle-aged mazes, and into her fabulous sixties.

For the juiciest tidbits about L's life, her "Manhattan Chronicles" blog is the place to be. This blog is an unfiltered dive into L's world, from her spiritual musings to her meticulous weigh-ins to her New Youniversity Chronicles—The Manhattan Diaries series—personal tales. Dive into her cosmos at her blog site: https://www.ManhattanChronicles.com.

The Manhattan Diaries Series

Eat Like an A-Lister
Manhattan's Ultimate Nutrition Guide

Manhattan Vitality
Just Like That

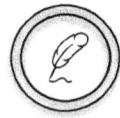

Introduction: Lights, Camera, Nutrition! – The Big Apple's Best-Kept A-Lister Secrets

Well, hello there, epicurean adventurers! As you navigate the dynamic culinary scene of Manhattan, have you ever wondered how the city's elite maintain their svelte figures while indulging in the gastronomic delights of the Big Apple? Do you strut through the city's culinary meccas with the confidence of a true New Yorker, or are you still decoding the secrets to eating like an A-lister in the city that never sleeps? Well, dear readers, the city's culinary world holds the key to ultimate nutrition, and I'm here to reveal it all in "Eat Like an A-Lister: Manhattan's Ultimate Nutrition Guide."

In this delectable journey, I'm taking you behind the scenes of Manhattan's discerning diners. Success in the Big Apple isn't just about wit or navigating the concrete jungle—it's about savoring cuisine that satisfies the palate and nourishes the body, all while maintaining a figure that's red carpet-ready. I've mingled with the city's culinary connoisseurs, indulged in exquisite dining experiences, and unearthed the nutrition secrets that keep Manhattan's finest feeling and looking their absolute best. But remember, true wellness begins from within.

Consider this your exclusive invitation to a limited-edition of The Manhattan Diaries series, culinary experience. Whether you savor this gastronomic treasure trove over leisurely meals, indulge in it week by week, or read it while sipping cocktails on Manhattan rooftops, the pace is entirely up to you. Visualize yourself diving into a chapter with your morning latte or immersing yourself in the entire book during a weekend foodie getaway. Within these pages, you'll unlock the keys to becoming the master of your nutrition destiny, and the vitality that follows will leave you feeling rejuvenated.

EAT LIKE AN A-LISTER

As we embark on this journey together, I'll be your culinary confidante, revealing how effortlessly you can dine like an A-lister in the city that never sleeps. This guide isn't just about nutrition tips: it's a revitalization of your spirit, your relationships, and your culinary aspirations in the city. Join me in uncovering the secrets that will allow you to savor every bite while maintaining the allure of a Manhattanite on the red carpet. I'm not just dedicated to helping you master the art of ultimate nutrition; I'm here to ignite the wellness in your heart that propels you to your most vibrant self. Embrace it, and the energy of New York will be yours to command!

My passion for this city-centric guide is born from my own personal journey, filled with culinary highs and lows, passion for food, and moments of culinary discovery. Like many city dwellers, I had to navigate the culinary maze, sometimes veering off the well-trodden path. But today, I stand before you, ready to inspire you to dine like an A-lister in the city, with a gourmet treat in hand.

As time sails on the Hudson River, our life paths inevitably intersect. For me the whirlwind of career pursuits, downtown culinary soirees, and self-discovery converged with my love for the city, leading me to work with the Urban Chronicles Publishing House.

New York City's culinary allure isn't limited to celebrities or trust fund beneficiaries; it's accessible to everyone, whether you're a gastronomic enthusiast in your twenties or a seasoned foodie in your sixties. Embrace this journey with me as we embark on a path to city stardom in this sixth step— The Manhattan Diaries series is a twenty-one step journey; twenty-one books to reinvent and discover a side of you Manhattan's never met.

"Eat Like an A-Lister" equips you with the tools to not only savor the best of the city's cuisine but also to maintain a figure that's red-carpet ready. I'm here as your city guardian, ensuring you realize that everything you crave starts within. Nourish your body with Manhattan's finest nutrition secrets, and watch as your wellness, vitality, and maybe even your dream partner, follow suit. If you've got culinary dreams of dining like an A-lister, this guide is your key to unlocking them! I've witnessed friends rise to nutritional stardom, proving that as you align within, the city will reflect it back in wellness and vitality. That's a promise straight from the heart of New York.

Relying on The Manhattan Diaries series has always been my compass. Whenever the city threw a culinary curveball my way, this guide, in The Manhattan Diaries series, steered me right back to my wellness path. The allure of always dining like an A-lister keeps me coming back to these pages, and trust me, it's far more exhilarating than settling for mediocrity.

With every page you turn, you'll discover the blueprint, insider secrets, and the support you need to make your journey an exhilarating adventure. This series is tailored for everyone, from those seeking a fabulous culinary career to social butterflies and food empire builders.

There are countless ways to rise in the Big Apple, but if you're looking for the chicest route to excellence, it's right here in The Manhattan Diaries. Immerse yourself in its treasures while reciting positive mantras, and let the city's vibrancy chase away any doubts; and, in this case, allowing you to dine like an A-lister and live your most vibrant life.

Navigating the City with The Manhattan Diaries

Welcome to "Eat Like an A-Lister: Manhattan's Ultimate Nutrition Guide." Think of this edition of The Manhattan Diaries as your personal cosmopolitan culinary diary, as interactive as an invitation to Manhattan's most exclusive gastronomic soirees. Each chapter is enriched with journal pages, waiting for your Manhattan musings and anecdotes. Whether you want to record the day's chic highlights in your "Culinary Chronicles" or delve into deep reflections in your "Culinary Confessions," these pages are yours to fill—see Cocktails and Chronicles: "Journal Pages: Pen Your Tales."

But . . .

1   Before you start penning your thoughts, take a moment to breathe. Close your eyes and, in that quiet moment, express a heartfelt "thank you" to the city that never sleeps. Feel that rush of gratitude, as if you've just been given a front row seat to a Michelin-starred culinary event. Let that "thank you" resonate deep within your heart—because that, my dear readers, is the magic of Manhattan.

2   Begin by detailing the fabulous strides you've made since delving into the last glamorous culinary advice you've received. Write them down under "Completed Tasks," and relish in the feeling of savoring every bite while maintaining your red-carpet allure.

3   Once you've celebrated your culinary triumphs, turn the page to "Action Items" and outline your gastronomic aspirations. Reflect on what's left to conquer in your culinary journey, capturing your next steps in this transformational saga.

Throughout The Manhattan Diaries series, you'll encounter timeless "inspirational quotes" that are as iconic as Manhattan's skyline. These pearls of wisdom are your city mantras. Get inspired by them, recite each word as if you're toasting at a chic restaurant, and let them resonate deep within your urban soul.

As you approach the end of each guide, you'll discover a "City Roundup." Here, you'll find a chic recap summarizing all the insider tips from your city escapade, ensuring you never miss a New York culinary minute.

So, get ready to dine like an A-lister, darlings. Behind the cityscape lies a world of culinary glamour, flavor, and endless possibilities for your palate. It's time to savor every bite and live your most epicurean life in the city that never sleeps.

LIGHTS, CAMERA, NUTRITION!

Eat Like an A-Lister: Manhattan's Ultimate Nutrition Guide

Darlings, picture this: the twinkling lights of Manhattan skyline, the click-clack of your Jimmy Choos, and a life filled with the vibrancy only Candace Bushnell can bring to words. Welcome to "Eat Like an A-Lister: Manhattan's Ultimate Nutrition Guide," the sixth seductive installment of The Manhattan Diaries series.

Every Carrie, Charlotte, Miranda, and Samantha knows there's an art to living large in the city of dreams. And honey, this isn't just about wearing the right shoes or attending the most fabulous parties. It's about the love affair with yourself! The way to the heart of this city? Through your stomach, and oh, the tantalizing tales I have for you.

Just two weeks. Give me a fortnight without the caffeinated temptations, the sugary sirens, and the alluring lull of alcohol. Swap them for lavish greens, sips of the purest H2O, and meals worthy of the red carpet. You'll not only glow differently, but darling, even your makeup drawer will take a sultry sigh of relief.

Step into the world of the A-listers, not just by dressing the part, but by dining with the grace and elegance of Manhattan's elite. Dive in, and discover the secrets to a life as sumptuous as a Manhattan penthouse view in "Eat Like an A-Lister: Manhattan's Ultimate Nutrition Guide."

Meet the Maestros Behind the Curtain

Welcome to the glittering realm of The Manhattan Diaries series, penned by an eclectic group of scribes who know how to make words shimmer just like that Midtown skyline. Each of these writers possesses the kind of Manhattan moxie that's as electrifying as a Saturday night at Studio 54. Picture the literary equivalent of the fabulous foursome from "Sex and the City," but with a little extra Manhattan mascara.

Our authors, darlings, aren't just writers; they're connoisseurs of all things NYC, dishing out stories with the precision of a Fifth Avenue stylist crafting the perfect blowout. Their tales are imbued with the kind of insider knowledge only those who've sipped martinis at the city's most secretive spots can truly understand.

So, as you delve into the pages of The Manhattan Diaries know that you're not just reading words, you're sipping on the prose of New York's finest literary mixologists. Here's to a journey as sparkling and unforgettable as a New York night out. Cheers, darling!

Behind the Scenes with the Urban Chronicles Publishing House

In the whirlwind of New York's high society, the Urban Chronicles Publishing House has emerged as the ultimate style sage for modern-day self-help. Over a cosmopolitan-fueled decade, they've become the city's go-to curators for crafting that sought-after, enviable life. The Manhattan Diaries? Envision it as your exclusive, VIP backstage pass, dripping with Upper East Side allure.

If you've ever pictured yourself sashaying through Manhattan with poise, if you've craved that skyline backdrop to your impeccable life, or if you simply seek the secrets whispered in the plush corners of the city's most exclusive clubs—The Manhattan Diaries is your ticket. Crafted under the elite banner, Urban Chronicles Publishing House, this imprint doesn't just offer you insights; it's your personal invite to the city's most glamorous circles.

- ➤ **Forever en Vogue**. Everyone, from the Wall Street moguls to the aspiring Broadway stars, dreams of basking in New York's radiant glow, of living a life drenched in style and substance. The wisdom in The Manhattan Diaries is as timeless as a Fifth Avenue romance, ensuring you're always en vogue.

➤ **A Blueprint for the Elite.** Nestled within these pages are the golden rules of city living, from mastering the cocktail chatter to undergoing a dazzling reinvention. Whether you're a seasoned socialite, an ambitious parent, or a fresh-eyed dreamer, these guides have something to make your heart race a little faster.

➤ **The Perfect Accessory.** Their petite stature makes these guides a seamless fit for your Prada clutch or your gym tote. Think of them as your urban survival kit—a blend of wisdom and wit that's as crucial as your red lipstick for those Manhattan nights.

Take a sip of this rich concoction, and let the Urban Chronicles Publishing House unlock Manhattan, unveiling a New York you only dreamed of. Welcome to the allure of the elite, darling.

Unveiling The Ridge Publishing Group

Picture The Ridge Publishing Group as the rising star on New York's literary and entertainment horizon. Envision an eclectic empire—books, cinema, and board games—setting the stage to become the world's haute couture of theological discourse. Think Fifth Avenue for theological resources: luxurious, elite, and unparalleled.

Dive into their esteemed collections. They hold the keys to the illustrious Guardians of Biblical Truth Publishing Group and the evocative New Narrated Study Bible (NNSB) series. Delve deeper and find the Hoyle Theology Publishing Group and its opulent Hoyle Theology Encyclopedia— a treasure trove for the cerebral sophisticate. And for those who like their theology paired with a cinematic flair, there's the Documentaries in Print Publishing Group with its tantalizing series like Defending the Faith. And, of course, for those cocktail nights with a side of divine strategy, the Heaven's Seminary board games and card decks offer a chic twist.

But that's not all. The Ridge Publishing Group is more than a theological publishing powerhouse; it's a brand. Alongside its flagship, it flaunts trendy imprints: AuthorsDoor Group and AuthorsDoor Leadership (check them out at the glamorous digital boulevard of https://www.AuthorsDoor.com), the ritzy Urban Chronicles Publishing House and New Youniversity (make your reservation at https://www.LAMoeszinger.com), and the novel delights of Ethan Fox Books (sip your martini and browse https://www.EthanFox Books.com).

For a sneak peek into the world where theology meets Manhattan glamour, rendezvous at their digital penthouse: https://www.Ridge PublishingGroup.com. It's theology made chic.

A NOTE TO THE READER

Typos in this book? Errors (and inconsistencies) can get through proofreaders, so if you do find any typos or grammatical errors in this book, I'd be very grateful if you could let me know using this email address typos@LAMoeszinger.com. Thank you ☺

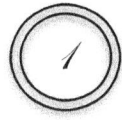

1

Uptown Greens:
Decoding the Salads of the Elite

Manhattan—a city that not only hears the clink of champagne flutes and the hum of high heels, but savors the subtle crunch of the freshest arugula and the tantalizing tang of a well-aged balsamic. In this urban jungle of ambitions and dreams, it isn't just about what you wear or where you're seen—it's about what you're seen eating. With panache, naturally.

Now picture this: You're seated at a sun-drenched bistro off Park Avenue, and as you delicately spear a vibrant leaf, every gaze is irresistibly pulled towards you. Not by the designer of your clutch, but by the artful composition of your plate. That darling, is the Manhattan Salad Sophistication, an elegance that whispers of culinary discernment and a palate that's truly in the know.

In this tantalizing chapter of The Manhattan Diaries, we'll journey into the leafy world of Uptown Greens. From the Caesar that's so passe to the frisée that's trés en vogue, you'll unravel the mysteries behind the salads that grace the tables of the city's crème de la crème.

But remember, this isn't just about greens and vinaigrettes. It's about understanding the intricate ballet of flavors and textures, a choreography that dances in harmony with the city's ever-evolving trends. It's about appreciating the sunlit terraces and the whispered deals they've witnessed, capturing the essence of Manhattan—one bite at a time.

So come along, as we savor the symphony of ingredients that make more than just a meal—they make a statement. Because, darling, in Manhattan, every forkful is an opportunity to dazzle. Ready your appetites and your aspirations, the city's salad secrets await our discovery. Welcome to The Manhattan Diaries—where your culinary choices can be as statement-making as the skyline itself.

The Salad Socialites

In the glittering playground of Manhattan's social elite, where Central Park picnics and Fifth Avenue shopping sprees intertwine seamlessly, there exists a delightful secret society: "The Salad Socialites." These tastemakers have mastered the art of turning greens into glamour, making salads the star of the show at every chic luncheon and soirée. Join me, darlings, as we peek behind the salad bowl curtain and delve into the lives of these salad aficionados who not only dine but truly define Manhattan's salad scene.

- ➤ **Salad Royalty at The Met**: Meet the queens and kings of the salad domain—the Upper East Side's salad royalty who have made greens their personal style statement, holding court in the elegant gardens of The Met.

- ➤ **Chic Salad Spots with Skyline Views**: Discover the exclusive restaurants and bistros where the socialites gather to see and be seen, all while indulging in the city's most fabulous salads, with sweeping skyline views from penthouse terraces.

- ➤ **Fashion on the Plate on Fifth Avenue**: Uncover the secrets of how these trendsetters pair their salads with the latest fashion trends, turning every meal into a runway show, as they stroll down Fifth Avenue in their finest couture.

- ➤ **Dressing to Impress at Tiffany's**: Explore the art of salad dressings and the custom creations that add a touch of sophistication to every bite, just like the exquisite jewels at Tiffany & Co.

- ➤ **Salad Soirées in Central Park**: Get an insider's look into the glamorous soirées and luncheons where the Salad Socialites showcase their culinary prowess amidst the lush greenery of Central Park, creating memories as timeless as The Plaza Hotel.

➤ **Big Apple-Inspired Creations**: Prepare to be delighted by the innovative salads that pay homage to iconic New York landmarks. Picture a towering skyscraper salad inspired by the Empire State Building, complete with crisp, vertical greens, or a Lady Liberty salad that boasts freedom-inspired ingredients, reminding us of the city's enduring spirit.

➤ **Salad on the Go**: From Cabs to Central Park: These socialites have mastered the art of enjoying salads on the go, whether it's relishing a classic Cobb salad during a yellow taxi ride through the bustling streets or savoring a Waldorf salad on a leisurely stroll through the enchanting landscapes of Central Park. Discover their secret to making salads a stylish, portable affair.

➤ **Salad Artistry that Rivals MoMA**: Step into the world of salad artistry, where plating techniques rival the creative genius found within the hallowed halls of the Museum of Modern Art. These Salad Socialites turn salads into edible masterpieces, crafting visually stunning compositions that are as captivating as the city's finest works of art.

➤ **Nightlife and Salad Suppers**: Join the Salad Socialites as they paint the town red and indulge in late-night salad suppers at exclusive clubs and bars, bringing a fresh twist to the city's bustling nightlife.

In the world of Manhattan's elite, it's not just about what you wear or where you're seen—it's about what's on your plate. And for "The Salad Socialites," every leaf, every ingredient is a canvas for their exquisite taste and style, weaving their stories into the iconic fabric of this city. So, prepare to be dazzled, dear readers, as we step into the captivating realm where salads are the stars, and every forkful is an opportunity to savor the high life in the city that never sleeps.

EAT LIKE AN A-LISTER

Completed Tasks: Salad Socialites Activities

Inspirational Quote

TRY OR CRY. CHOOSE! — Heenashree Khandelwal

UPTOWN GREENS

Action Items: Intentions and Thoughts

EAT LIKE AN A-LISTER

From Cobb to Kale

In the ever-evolving culinary landscape of Manhattan, where trends and tastes shift as swiftly as a Fifth Avenue fashion show, the story of salads is a testament to the city's dynamic spirit. From the classic Cobb salad to the kale craze that's taken Manhattan by storm, the salad scene here is a journey of transformation and reinvention. Join me, darlings, as we embark on a delectable exploration of "From Cobb to Kale," tracing the trajectory of these greens from timeless classics to the trendiest plates, all while weaving in the iconic landmarks that make Manhattan the vibrant heart of gastronomic innovation.

- ➢ **The Cobb Salad: A Classic Born at the Waldorf:** Let's start our journey with a classic-the legendary Cobb salad. Born at the historic Waldorf Astoria, this timeless ensemble of chicken, bacon, and avocado has been a staple on Manhattan menus for decades.

- ➢ **Kale: The Green Queen of Manhattan**: Explore the kale phenomenon that has swept across Manhattan, gracing the plates of health-conscious New Yorkers. This leafy superstar has become synonymous with vitality and can be found everywhere, from trendy SoHo eateries to bustling Midtown cafes.

- ➢ **New York Reimagined: The Art of Salad Transformation**: Dive into the creative minds behind the salad revolution. Manhattan's innovative chefs and culinary wizards have taken salads to new heights, fusing diverse flavors and ingredients to create unique masterpieces that redefine the concept of a salad.

- ➢ **Landmarks on the Plate**: As we traverse this culinary journey, we'll intertwine the salad evolution with iconic Manhattan landmarks. Imagine savoring a kale salad with Central Park views or relishing a Cobb salad at a charming eatery near Times Square-the city's landmarks serve as a backdrop to our gastronomic adventure.

➢ **Rooftop Revelations: Elevated Salad Experiences**: Ascend to Manhattan's chic rooftop bars and restaurants where salads have reached new heights—both literally and figuratively. Savor the fresh flavors of kale and other greens while enjoying breathtaking views of the Empire State Building and the city's iconic skyscrapers.

➢ **Street Eats & Food Trucks**: Kale Takes to the Streets: Manhattan's bustling streets are home to an array of food trucks and street vendors offering inventive kale-based creations that satisfy both the hurried New Yorker and the curious tourist. Join us on a culinary tour of the city's sidewalk sensations.

➢ **Salad Sourcing Secrets**: Delve into the secrets of sourcing the freshest ingredients in the concrete jungle. Discover how Manhattan's chefs maintain their commitment to quality and sustainability in the midst of the city's hustle, with visits to local markets like Union Square Greenmarket and Chelsea Market.

➢ **Cocktail Couture: Pairing Salads with Signature Sips**: Explore the art of pairing salads with signature cocktails at Manhattan's trendiest bars and lounges. Experience the fusion of flavors as mixologists craft kale-inspired concoctions that perfectly complement the salad scene, all while enjoying the glitz and glamour of nightlife along the iconic Broadway.

In the ever-changing cityscape of NYC, where the skyline is a canvas and every street corner tells a story, salads have undergone a metamorphosis. From the classic Cobb's inception at the Waldorf Astoria to kale's reign as the Green Queen, Manhattan's salad scene is a testament to the city's ability to embrace change while staying true to its iconic character. So, stay tuned, dear readers, as we continue to unravel the salad evolution amidst the backdrop of Manhattan's most beloved landmarks, where every bite is a taste of innovation and a tribute to the city that never ceases to amaze.

EAT LIKE AN A-LISTER

Completed Tasks: From Cobb to Kale Activities

Inspirational Quote

WHEN YOU FOCUS ON BEING THE BEST PERSON YOU CAN BE, YOU DRAW
THE BEST POSSIBLE LIFE, LOVE, AND OPPORTUNITIES TO YOU. — Germany
Kent

UPTOWN GREENS

Action Items: Intentions and Thoughts

The Art of Salad Pairings: From Greens to Grapes

In the chic world of Manhattan's culinary elite, where every meal is a performance, there exists an art form that elevates dining to a symphony of flavors: the art of salad pairings. From the delicate interplay of greens and vinaigrettes to the harmonious fusion of ingredients with fine wines, these salad aficionados have mastered the exquisite dance between greens and grapes. Join me, darlings, as we delve into "The Art of Salad Pairings: From Greens to Grapes," where every bite is a tantalizing sip of sophistication, intertwined with the iconic landmarks that define the Manhattan dining experience.

➢ **Green Symphony: The Perfect Salad and Wine Harmony**: Step into the world of gastronomic elegance as we explore the timeless pairing of salads with the finest wines. Discover the secrets behind matching the right salad with the perfect vintage, transforming every dining experience into a work of art.

➢ **Vineyard to Table: Exploring Manhattan's Wine Scene**: Embark on a wine-tasting adventure through Manhattan's wine bars and cellars, where sommeliers curate exquisite selections that complement the city's diverse salad offerings. From the enchanting Upper West Side to the lively Lower East Side, each neighborhood boasts its unique wine destinations.

➢ **The Met Gala of Pairings: Gourmet Salad Extravaganzas**: Experience exclusive soirées and gourmet gatherings where the city's culinary elite showcase their expertise in salad pairings. Picture sipping a Chardonnay at a rooftop garden event overlooking Central Park or enjoying a Pinot Noir amidst the opulence of a Midtown gala.

➢ **Iconic Settings for Culinary Artistry**: As we journey through Manhattan's gastronomic wonders, we'll intertwine the art of salad pairings with the city's iconic landmarks. Imagine savoring a perfectly paired salad and wine duo against the backdrop of the historic Flatiron Building or the majestic Brooklyn Bridge, where history and culinary innovation unite.

➢ **Farm-to-Table Salad Alchemy**: Explore the farm-to-table movement in Manhattan's dining scene, where chefs collaborate with local farmers to create seasonal salad masterpieces that perfectly complement the region's wines. From the Union Square Greenmarket to the High Line's artisanal vendors, discover the freshness of locally sourced ingredients.

➢ **Champagne Dreams and Salad Realities**: Unveil the secrets of pairing salads with champagne, an epitome of luxury dining. Join Manhattan's elite as they indulge in effervescent pairings amidst the opulent ambiance of the Plaza Hotel's Champagne Bar or the timeless glamour of the Rainbow Room at Rockefeller Center.

➢ **Salad Culture in Iconic Neighborhoods**: Discover the unique salad culture in Manhattan's iconic neighborhoods, from the Upper East Side's classic charm to the trendy vibes of Williamsburg. Each neighborhood's culinary scene reflects its character and history, offering diverse salad pairings that pay homage to their heritage.

In the realm of Manhattan's elite, every meal is a statement, and these salad pairings are a testament to the city's commitment to culinary artistry. From the perfect salad and wine harmony to exploring the city's vibrant wine scene and indulging in gourmet salad extravaganzas, this is a world where flavors and finesse come together in perfect union. So, stay tuned, dear readers, as we continue to uncover the artistry of salad pairings amidst the backdrop of Manhattan's timeless landmarks, where every bite and sip is a masterpiece in the heart of the city that never sleeps.

Completed Tasks: Salad Pairings Activities

Inspirational Quote

LIFE IS HALF SPENT BEFORE WE KNOW WHAT IT IS. — George Herbert

Action Items: Intentions and Thoughts

Secrets of the Salad Dressing: Unmasking Manhattan's Hidden Flavor Gems

In the vibrant tapestry of Manhattan's dining scene, where every bite is an exploration of flavor and finesse, there exists a hidden world of culinary intrigue: the secrets of salad dressings. Beyond the greens and ingredients lies the art of crafting the perfect dressing, a symphony of flavors that elevate salads to new heights. Join me, darlings, as we delve into "Secrets of the Salad Dressing: Unmasking Manhattan's Hidden Flavor Gems," where we'll unmask the hidden treasures that make salads unforgettable, all while weaving in the iconic landmarks that define the city's culinary landscape.

➢ **The Dressing Revelation: Beyond the Vinaigrettes:** Step into the dressing room of Manhattan's salad scene, where we'll uncover the creativity of chefs who go beyond traditional vinaigrettes. Discover the secrets behind creamy avocado dressings, tantalizing truffle-infused oils, and exotic miso-based concoctions that add depth and character to every bite.

➢ **Chef's Signature Dressings**: Explore the culinary alchemy of Manhattan's top chefs as they reveal their signature dressings. Imagine indulging in a salad dressed with Daniel Boulud's legendary mustard vinaigrette or Jean-Georges Vongerichten's innovative ginger-miso blend, where each dressing is a work of art in itself.

➢ **Market Fresh and Locally Sourced Dressings**: Experience the farm-to-table movement in salad dressings, where locally sourced and market-fresh ingredients are used to create dressings that capture the essence of Manhattan's diverse neighborhoods. From the bustling markets of Union Square to the artisanal vendors along the High Line, discover the magic of freshness.

➢ **Dressing & Mixology: The Cocktail Connection**: Unveil the connection between salad dressings and mixology, where innovative mixologists craft cocktails inspired by salad dressings. Sip on a cocktail that mirrors the flavors of your salad dressing at trendy bars like PDT (Please Don't Tell) or the speakeasy-style Angel's Share.

➤ **Sweet Surrender: Dessert Dressings and Toppings**: Explore the enchanting world of dessert dressings and toppings that transform salads into delectable sweets. Indulge in Manhattan's unique dessert salad creations, where dressings infused with honey, caramel, and balsamic reductions turn salads into heavenly treats, much like the sumptuous desserts at Serendipity 3.

➤ **Citrus Infusion: Zest and Zing**: Immerse yourself in the zesty and refreshing world of citrus-infused dressings. Discover how Manhattan's chefs use lemon, lime, and orange zest to add brightness and a burst of flavor to their salads, reminiscent of the vibrant energy of Times Square.

➤ **Fresh Herb Elegance**: Delve into the elegance of fresh herb dressings that elevate salads to new heights. From basil-infused dressings reminiscent of a stroll through the serene Central Park Conservatory Garden to minty creations that evoke the charm of the West Village's tree-lined streets, these dressings are a tribute to nature's bounty.

In the world of Manhattan's elite dining, where every dish is a revelation and every dressing holds a secret, the journey through the hidden flavor gems of salad dressings is a testament to the city's culinary innovation. As we continue our exploration, dear readers, remember that Manhattan's iconic landmarks are not just a backdrop but an integral part of the city's vibrant culinary tapestry. Stay tuned for more unmasking of Manhattan's salad dressing secrets, where each bite is a taste of history and a tribute to the city that never ceases to surprise and delight.

EAT LIKE AN A-LISTER

Completed Tasks: Salad Dressing Secrets Activities

UPTOWN GREENS

Action Items: Intentions and Thoughts

Salads with a View: Manhattan's Most Glamorous Al Fresco Dining

In the glamorous world of Manhattan's elite, where every meal is an opportunity to see and be seen, al fresco dining with a view takes center stage. Amidst the city's iconic landmarks and glittering skyscrapers, open-air terraces and rooftop gardens offer a taste of the high life, where salads become a sophisticated statement against a backdrop of Manhattan's breathtaking vistas. Join me, darlings, as we explore "Salads with a View: Manhattan's Most Glamorous Al Fresco Dining," where every bite is an enchanting experience, intertwined with the city's timeless landmarks that define Manhattan's skyline.

➢ **Rooftop Reverie: Skyline Salad Soirees**: Ascend to Manhattan's chic rooftop bars and restaurants, where the city's elite gather for skyline salad soirees. Picture savoring a kale Caesar salad while overlooking the sparkling lights of Times Square or enjoying a classic Cobb salad with Central Park as your backdrop.

➢ **Parkside Pleasures: Central Park Picnics**: Experience the enchantment of picnics in Central Park, where salad connoisseurs indulge in gourmet greens amidst the lush greenery and serene lakes. Imagine enjoying a Waldorf salad while lounging near Bethesda Terrace or sharing a quinoa salad with friends by the iconic Bow Bridge.

➢ **Skyscraper Suppers: Dining Amongst Giants**: Dine amidst the giants of the concrete jungle at exclusive restaurants that offer al fresco dining with a view of Manhattan's iconic skyscrapers. Enjoy a frisée salad with a glimpse of the Empire State Building at the renowned Gramercy Tavern or relish a Caprese salad while marveling at One World Trade Center's majesty.

➢ **Terrace Tales: Outdoor Gardens and Hidden Oases**: Explore the secret gardens and hidden terraces that dot Manhattan's landscape, providing a peaceful escape from the city's hustle and bustle. Picture yourself savoring a Mediterranean salad in the enchanting garden of Maison Premiere in Williamsburg or enjoying a rooftop frisée salad at the charming Bar Six in the West Village.

➢ **Wine and Dine by the Hudson**: Immerse yourself in the romantic atmosphere of al fresco dining along the Hudson River. Discover the joy of pairing your salad with fine wines while gazing at the water's edge, where the George Washington Bridge stands as a magnificent backdrop.

➢ **Highline Haven: Elevated Salad Retreats**: Explore the charm of dining on the High Line, Manhattan's elevated park with stunning views of the city and the Hudson River. Enjoy a salad while strolling amidst wildflowers and contemporary art installations, soaking in the ambiance of this unique urban oasis.

➢ **Riverside Revelations: East River Magic**: Savor the magic of dining by the East River, where you can indulge in seafood-inspired salads with views of the Brooklyn Bridge and the Manhattan skyline. Imagine the delight of a lobster salad while basking in the glow of the city's shimmering lights.

As we traverse the glamorous al fresco dining scene of Manhattan, where salads become a culinary experience against the city's iconic landmarks, remember that these outdoor settings are more than just dining spaces—they are a reflection of the city's ever-evolving trends and the vibrant spirit that defines Manhattan. Stay tuned, dear readers, for more revelations of al fresco dining with a view, where each bite and every vista is a testament to the city's timeless allure and the remarkable stories it continues to tell.

Completed Tasks: Salads with a View Activities

Inspirational Quote

LET EACH MAN EXERCISE THE ART HE KNOWS. — Aristophanes

UPTOWN GREENS

Action Items: Intentions and Thoughts

Action Items: Intentions and Thoughts

2

Madison Avenue Munchies:
Snacking with Style and Substance

Manhattan—a city where every crumb tells a tale, where each nibble is imbued with narratives of passion, purpose, and a dash of panache. In the city that never sleeps, it's not merely about satisfying hunger, but about feeding the soul with snacks that are both delectable and distinguished.

Now, envision this: You're strolling past the illustrious shop windows on Madison Avenue, each bite you take is met with intrigued glances. Not because of the brand adorning your wrist, but due to the chic morsel you're effortlessly enjoying. That, darling, is the Madison Avenue Munchie Magic—a gastronomic gesture that's equal parts allure and assertion.

In this delightful chapter of The Manhattan Diaries, we'll delve into the art of snacking in style. From the daintiest macarons that melt on the tongue to the bold, savory bites that announce one's arrival, we'll explore how to satiate with substance and swagger.

But remember, this isn't solely about savoring flavors. It's about the dance of textures and tastes that embody the essence of the metropolis, about choosing snacks that tell a tale of discernment, ambition, and a hint of audacity. It's about being in sync with the city's heartbeat, its vibrant rhythms and its quiet pauses.

So, join me, as we embark on a culinary sojourn, unveiling the secrets of snacks that not only appease the appetite but command attention. For in Manhattan, even the tiniest treat is an expression of one's taste. Lace up those stilettos and set your senses alight, for the city's waiting to share its snacking secrets. Welcome to The Manhattan Diaries—where even your munchies can echo the grandeur of Gotham.

The Snacking Socialites: A Bite with the Elite

In the glittering social tapestry of Manhattan, where each nibble becomes an opportunity to see and be seen, there exists a cadre of epicurean elite known as the "Snacking Socialites." These tastemakers and trendsetters have turned the art of snacking into a chic affair that combines sophistication with delectable bites. Join me, darlings, as we step into the world of "The Snacking Socialites," where every snack is a culinary statement, and style knows no bounds. Here are the enticing bullet points to whet your appetite:

> **Snacking in the Spotlight:** Explore the allure of snacking in the city, where every bite becomes an act of gastronomic theatre, and the Snacking Socialites are the stars of the show.

> **The Power of Presentation:** Delve into the art of presentation, where snacks are not just delectable but also visually stunning. Discover how the Snacking Socialites elevate their snacking game with elegant plating and presentation.

> **Exclusive Snack Soirées:** Get an exclusive peek into the world of snack soirées, where the elite gather to nibble on gourmet bites and sip on the finest champagne. Imagine attending a rooftop macaron and champagne soiree overlooking the iconic Flatiron Building.

> **Nightlife and Nibbles:** Explore the vibrant nightlife scene where the Snacking Socialites indulge in late-night snacks at swanky bars and lounges. Picture savoring truffle fries and craft cocktails amidst the glitz and glamour of Broadway.

> **Manhattan's Culinary Landmarks:** As we journey through the Snacking Socialites' world, we'll intertwine their snacking adventures with Manhattan's iconic landmarks. Imagine enjoying a gourmet hot dog near the Empire State Building or sipping on espresso martinis in the shadow of the Chrysler Building.

- ➤ **High Tea Extravaganzas**: Delight in the tradition of high tea with a Manhattan twist as we explore the Snacking Socialites' penchant for luxurious tea parties. Picture indulging in delicate finger sandwiches and exquisite pastries in the opulent setting of The Plaza Hotel's Palm Court.

- ➤ **Global Snacking Escapades**: Join the Snacking Socialites on their globetrotting snacking escapades as they explore international flavors without leaving Manhattan. From Japanese-inspired sushi bites in the heart of Little Tokyo to exotic Middle Eastern mezze at a hidden gem in the West Village, discover how they bring the world to their plates.

- ➤ **Art and Appetizers**: Immerse yourself in the intersection of art and culinary creativity as we visit gallery openings and exhibitions that pair exquisite appetizers with artistic flair. Imagine savoring gourmet hors d'oeuvres at a contemporary art gallery in Chelsea, where every bite is a work of art.

- ➤ **Rooftop Garden Feasts**: Experience the Snacking Socialites' rooftop garden feasts, where they dine amidst lush greenery and city views. Picture relishing seasonal snacks made from rooftop-grown ingredients while gazing at the iconic skyline, with the Freedom Tower as a backdrop.

In Manhattan, darling, even the smallest bite is an opportunity to shine, and the Snacking Socialites have mastered the art of making their snacks as chic as the Upper East Side boutiques. These culinary stars have turned snacking into a glamorous affair, leaving their mark on the city's gastronomic landscape. Stay tuned, dear readers, as we continue to unravel the world of the Snacking Socialites amidst the iconic landmarks of Manhattan, where every bite and every glimpse is a taste of elegance and a tribute to the city that never ceases to inspire.

Completed Tasks: Snacking Socialites Activities

Inspirational Quote

TODAY IS THE ONLY DAY. YESTERDAY IS GONE. — John Wooden

Action Items: Intentions and Thoughts

Macarons and Munchies: Delicate Bites that Dazzle

In the glittering culinary landscape of Manhattan, where every bite is a chance to make a statement, one category of snacks stands out with its delicate allure and irresistible charm: macarons and munchies. These petite, exquisite treats have the power to dazzle the senses and elevate any snacking experience to a higher level of sophistication. Join me, darlings, as we delve into the world of "Macarons and Munchies: Delicate Bites that Dazzle," where every nibble is an artful indulgence, intertwined with the iconic landmarks that define the Manhattan dining scene.

➢ **The Macaron Magic**: Step into the enchanting world of macarons, those delicate, pastel-hued confections that are a symbol of elegance and refinement. Explore the artistry behind crafting these almond meringue delights and how they have become a culinary status symbol in Manhattan's high society.

➢ **High Tea Elegance**: Join us for a tea party fit for Manhattan royalty as we explore the tradition of high tea with a modern twist. Discover the delightful pairings of macarons with fine teas and finger sandwiches in iconic tea rooms like The Russian Tea Room, where history and taste intertwine.

➢ **Gourmet Gelato and Sorbet**: Venture into the world of gourmet gelato and sorbet, where the Snacking Socialites indulge in flavors that go beyond the ordinary. Imagine savoring a scoop of blood orange sorbet with a view of the Manhattan Bridge from a charming gelateria in DUMBO.

➢ **Landmarks of Sweet Temptation**: As we savor these delightful delicacies, we'll also intertwine our journey with Manhattan's iconic landmarks. Picture enjoying macarons while strolling through Central Park's Bethesda Terrace or sipping on an affogato with views of the Brooklyn Bridge at a DUMBO cafe.

➢ **Artisanal Chocolates**: Explore the world of artisanal chocolates and truffles, where each piece is a work of art. Join the Snacking Socialites as they visit boutique chocolate shops in the West Village, savoring handcrafted chocolates that mirror the creativity of Manhattan's art galleries.

➢ **Honeycomb Bliss**: Indulge in the luxurious world of honeycomb-inspired desserts, where golden honey drizzles over delicate bites. Picture tasting honey-infused macarons and baklava while sipping on artisanal honey cocktails at a rooftop bar overlooking the Hudson River.

➢ **Pâtisserie Perfection**: Discover the pâtisseries that elevate dessert to a form of art. Explore the artful creations of Manhattan's renowned pastry chefs, from éclairs that pay homage to the Guggenheim Museum to petit fours that capture the essence of Broadway.

➢ **Snacking at Iconic Lounges**: Immerse yourself in the ambiance of iconic lounges and jazz clubs where macarons and elegant snacks are the perfect accompaniments to live music. Imagine sipping on a cocktail at the Blue Note Jazz Club while enjoying a platter of French macarons.

In Manhattan, darling, even the smallest bite is a chance to indulge in luxury, and macarons and munchies have become the epitome of indulgence. These delicate bites have the power to transport us to a world of elegance and charm, all against the backdrop of the city's iconic landmarks. Stay tuned, dear readers, as we continue to explore the world of macarons and munchies amidst the grandeur of Manhattan, where every nibble and every vista is a testament to the city's timeless allure and its ability to make every moment a celebration of style and taste.

Completed Tasks: Macarons and Munchies Activities

Action Items: Intentions and Thoughts

Savory Swagger: Bold and Flavorful Bites

In the heart of Manhattan's vibrant dining scene, where boldness is celebrated and flavor is king, there exists a world of snacks that exude "Savory Swagger." These bites make a statement, announcing one's arrival with an audacious burst of taste that leaves an indelible mark. Join me, darlings, as we embark on a journey into "Savory Swagger: Bold and Flavorful Bites," where every nibble is a declaration of culinary confidence, intertwined with the iconic landmarks that define Manhattan's spirited dining culture.

➢ **The Art of Gourmet Burgers**: Enter the realm of gourmet burgers, where chefs push the boundaries of flavor with innovative creations. Discover how Manhattan's Snacking Socialites indulge in towering burgers with foie gras or truffle-infused patties, transforming the humble burger into a gourmet masterpiece.

➢ **Tantalizing Tacos and Street Eats**: Immerse yourself in the world of street eats and tantalizing tacos as we explore the diverse flavors of Manhattan's food trucks and pop-up stalls. Picture savoring spicy Korean BBQ tacos at Madison Square Park or enjoying Venezuelan arepas in the vibrant East Village.

➢ **Pizza with Pizzazz**: Join us on a pizza pilgrimage to Manhattan's top pizzerias, where bold flavors and inventive toppings reign supreme. Imagine indulging in a slice of truffle and mushroom pizza at a historic pizzeria in Little Italy or relishing a Roman-style pizza with skyline views at a rooftop pizza joint.

➢ **Sushi Sensations**: Dive into the world of sushi and sashimi, where the Snacking Socialites embark on culinary adventures with the freshest seafood. Explore the art of omakase dining at a hidden sushi gem in Tribeca or indulge in sushi rolls that pay homage to Broadway's musicals.

- ➢ **Manhattan's Culinary Landmarks**: As we savor these bold and flavorful bites, we'll intertwine our journey with Manhattan's iconic landmarks. Picture enjoying a gourmet burger in the shadow of the Flatiron Building or relishing street tacos near the historic Stonewall Inn.

- ➢ **Fried Chicken Frenzy**: Indulge in the irresistible world of fried chicken, where crispy, juicy bites are celebrated in their many forms. Join the Snacking Socialites as they embark on fried chicken crawls across Harlem, relishing iconic dishes that pay homage to the neighborhood's rich culinary heritage.

- ➢ **Spice and Heat Adventures**: Explore the fiery flavors of Manhattan's spicy cuisine, where bold spices and heat take center stage. Picture yourself indulging in Szechuan hot pot in Chinatown or savoring spicy tacos in East Harlem, where every bite is a journey into the heart of flavor.

- ➢ **International Dumpling Delights**: Delve into the global world of dumplings, where cultures converge and flavors unite. Join in a quest for the perfect dumpling, whether it's Japanese gyoza in the East Village or Polish pierogi on the Lower East Side.

- ➢ **Bites and Brews**: Discover the art of pairing bold bites with craft beers at Manhattan's top breweries and gastropubs.

In Manhattan, darling, even the most casual snack is an opportunity to make a statement and showcase culinary prowess. These bold and flavorful bites reflect the city's ever-evolving dining culture and are often enjoyed against the backdrop of its iconic landmarks. Stay tuned, dear readers, as we continue to explore the world of "Savory Swagger" amidst the grandeur of Gotham, where every bite and every view is a testament to the city's vibrant spirit and the remarkable stories it continues to tell.

Completed Tasks: Savory Swagger Activities

Action Items: Intentions and Thoughts

Snacking with Substance: The Narrative of Nourishment

In the labyrinthine streets of Manhattan, where every culinary choice is a statement and every bite tells a story, there exists a movement among the elite known as "Snacking with Substance." These tastemakers have turned the act of snacking into an opportunity to nourish not only their appetites but also their consciences, all while making a stylish mark on the city's dining scene. Join me, darlings, as we delve into "Snacking with Substance: The Narrative of Nourishment," where every nibble carries a purpose, intertwined with the iconic landmarks that define the Manhattan dining culture.

- ➤ **The Rise of Sustainable Snacking**: Explore the world of sustainable snacking, where the Snacking Socialites choose bites that align with their commitment to eco-conscious living. Picture enjoying organic, locally sourced snacks while supporting farmer's markets near Union Square or indulging in plant-based options that celebrate the vitality of Battery Park's urban gardens.

- ➤ **Healthy Bites on the Go**: Venture into the realm of wholesome, on-the-go snacks that nourish both body and soul. Join us as we discover the Snacking Socialites' favorite spots for nutrient-packed smoothie bowls in Chelsea Market or sampling organic energy bars at pop-up health food stands in Midtown.

- ➤ **Culinary Philanthropy**: Delve into the world of culinary philanthropy, where dining choices are guided by a commitment to social responsibility. Imagine attending charity events at prestigious venues like The Metropolitan Museum of Art, where exquisite hors d'oeuvres are created by renowned chefs in support of important causes.

- ➤ **Manhattan's Culinary Landmarks**: As we savor these snacks with substance, well intertwine our journey with Manhattan's iconic landmarks. Picture enjoying a vegan street food feast in the heart of Greenwich Village's Washington Square Park or participating in a charity walk along the Hudson River Park's scenic trails.

➤ **Farm-to-Table Experiences**: Immerse yourself in the farm-to-table movement, where the Snacking Socialites support restaurants that prioritize locally sourced, seasonal ingredients. Imagine dining at a charming West Village eatery where the menu is inspired by the Union Square Greenmarket, or relishing a rooftop dinner with panoramic views of the Hudson River, featuring sustainable seafood and vegetables grown on-site.

➤ **Community Culinary Initiatives**: Explore the world of community-based culinary initiatives where dining choices are intertwined with community support. Join the Snacking Socialites in participating in soup kitchens and food drives at iconic locations like The Bowery Mission, where generosity is as much a part of the dining experience as the flavors themselves.

➤ **Urban Picnics with a Purpose**: Embrace the joy of urban picnics in Manhattan's parks, where the Snacking Socialites gather for stylish outdoor feasts. Imagine joining them for a Central Park picnic featuring a spread of sustainable sandwiches and organic salads, all while surrounded by the park's lush greenery and iconic landmarks.

In the world of "Snacking with Substance," every bite is a declaration of values and a celebration of purpose, all set against the backdrop of Manhattan's iconic landmarks. As we continue our exploration, dear readers, remember that these landmarks aren't just scenery but integral components of the dining experience, where every nibble and every vista is a testament to the city's commitment to making the world a better place and the remarkable stories it continues to tell. Stay tuned for more revelations of conscious dining amidst the grandeur of Gotham.

Completed Tasks: Snacking with Substance Activities

_____

_____

_____

_____

_____

_____

_____

_____

_____

_____

_____

_____

_____

_____

_____

_____

_____

_____

_____

_____

_____

_____

_____

_____

_____

_____

_____

_____

_____

_____

_____

_____

_____

Inspirational Quote

PRAYER IS MAN'S GREATEST POWER! — W. Clement Stone

Action Items: Intentions and Thoughts

Madison Avenue Moments: The Art of Snacking in Style

In the glittering world of Manhattan's Madison Avenue, where style reigns supreme, every snacking moment is a chance to make a statement. It's a place where the chicest morsels are enjoyed with flair, and the act of snacking becomes an art form in itself. Join me, darlings, as we delve into "Madison Avenue Moments: The Art of Snacking in Style," where every nibble is a reflection of impeccable taste, intertwined with the iconic landmarks that define the Manhattan social scene.

➤ **Champagne and Canapés**: Embark on a journey into the world of champagne and canapés, where the Snacking Socialites indulge in the finest bubbles and gourmet bite-sized creations. Picture sipping on Dom Pérignon while nibbling on caviar-topped blinis at a chic Madison Avenue salon.

➤ **Afternoon Tea Elegance**: Explore the tradition of afternoon tea with a modern twist at Manhattan's iconic tea salons. Discover how the Snacking Socialites revel in the grandeur of The St. Regis New York's King Cole Bar with its legendary Bloody Mary and tea sandwiches or savoring high tea with skyline views at The Peninsula New York.

➤ **Artful Tapas and Small Plates**: Immerse yourself in the world of artful tapas and small plates at Manhattan's trendiest tapas bars. Imagine dining on a rooftop with views of the Empire State Building while enjoying a selection of creative small plates inspired by the city's diverse neighborhoods.

➤ **Cocktails and Charcuterie**: Join us as we explore the pairing of cocktails with charcuterie boards at Manhattan's chic lounges and speakeasies. Picture sipping on classic cocktails while indulging in a selection of artisanal cheeses and cured meats in the hidden corners of the West Village.

➤ **Manhattan's Culinary Landmarks**: As we savor these stylish snacks, we'll intertwine our journey with Manhattan's iconic landmarks. Picture enjoying a lavish champagne brunch at Tavern on the Green in Central Park or relishing afternoon tea at The Met Cloisters, surrounded by medieval art and serene gardens.

➤ **Dessert and Design**: Immerse yourself in the world of dessert and design at Manhattan's most stylish patisseries and dessert boutiques. Join the Snacking Socialites as they indulge in designer desserts inspired by the latest fashion trends, such as edible handbag-shaped pastries and high-heeled shoe chocolates.

➤ **Mixology Masterpieces**: Explore the art of mixology at upscale cocktail bars, where the Snacking Socialites enjoy bespoke cocktails paired with inventive snacks. Imagine sipping on a Manhattan-inspired cocktail while nibbling on truffle popcorn at a bar overlooking the Flatiron Building.

➤ **Sushi Couture**: Dive into the world of sushi couture, where the Snacking Socialites experience sushi as a work of art. Discover the artistry of sushi chefs who craft exquisite, jewel-like nigiri and sashimi, transforming a meal into a visual and culinary masterpiece.

In Manhattan, darling, even the smallest bite is a chance to indulge in luxury, and Madison Avenue is the epicenter of snacking in style. These Madison Avenue moments reflect the city's dedication to elegance and impeccable taste, all set against the backdrop of its iconic landmarks. Stay tuned, dear readers, as we continue to explore the world of snacking in style amidst the grandeur of Gotham, where every bite and every view is a testament to the city's timeless allure and the remarkable stories it continues to tell.

Completed Tasks: Snacking in Style Activities

Action Items: Intentions and Thoughts

Action Items: Intentions and Thoughts

3

Central Park Picnics:
Alfresco Dining with a Gourmet Twist

Manhattan—a city where skyscrapers rise high and dreams soar even higher, where every meal is not just a mere act of eating but a performance to be celebrated. And amidst the city's symphony of hustle and haste, there lies an oasis where gourmet dreams take flight under the open sky: Central Park.

Imagine this: You're elegantly sprawled on the verdant lawns, with the Manhattan skyline as your backdrop. Every passerby stops and stares, not because of the designer label on your picnic blanket, but the finesse with which you've orchestrated an alfresco feast. Sweetheart, that's the Central Park Picnic Panache—a culinary performance that resonates with elegance, eclecticism, and an edge of the unexpected.

In this gourmet chapter of The Manhattan Diaries, we'll whisk you away into the world of posh picnics. From exquisitely marinated olives that spark tales of distant lands to artisanal cheeses that dance with both depth and daring, you'll learn to lay out a spread that's the talk of the town.

But it's not just about the food. It's about setting a stage amidst nature, allowing the gentle rustle of leaves and the subtle chirps to serenade you. It's about juxtaposing the urban and the natural, relishing in the romance of Manhattan's green heart while also making a statement that's distinctively Upper East Side.

So, come along, as we saunter through sunlit pathways and hidden alcoves, crafting an outdoor dining experience that's as much about the ambiance as the flavors. Because, darling, in Manhattan, every picnic is an opportunity to showcase style, substance, and a dash of spontaneity. Uncork that bubbly and spread out that charcuterie, for Central Park beckons. Welcome to The Manhattan Diaries—where your picnic can be as legendary as a New York minute.

EAT LIKE AN A-LISTER

Picnic Perfection

In the enchanting realm of Central Park, where the city's heartbeat harmonizes with nature's tranquility, one art takes center stage: "Picnic Perfection." These outdoor feasts are not just about savoring exquisite flavors; they're performances of culinary finesse, transforming picnicking into a symphony of style. Join me, darlings, as we delve into "Picnic Perfection," where every element, from the choice of the picnic blanket to the arrangement of gourmet delights, is meticulously orchestrated, all while weaving in the iconic landmarks that define the Manhattan landscape.

➢ **Blanket Chic**: Discover the art of selecting the perfect picnic blanket that complements your style and sets the stage for a gourmet alfresco experience. Explore the Snacking Socialites' favorite spots for handcrafted, designer picnic blankets that evoke the essence of Manhattan's chic elegance.

➢ **Gourmet Grazing**: Indulge in the world of gourmet grazing, where the Snacking Socialites curate picnic menus that rival the finest restaurants. Imagine savoring dishes like truffle-infused lobster rolls and champagne-drenched strawberries amidst the lush foliage of Central Park's iconic Bethesda Terrace.

➢ **Wines and Whimsy**: Explore the pairing of wines with whimsical picnic fare at Manhattan's most picturesque picnic spots. Picture sipping on a velvety Pinot Noir while nibbling on gourmet charcuterie near the iconic Bow Bridge, creating a harmonious fusion of flavors and vistas.

➢ **Nature's Backdrop**: Delve into the magic of Central Park's natural beauty, where hidden alcoves and sunlit glades become the canvas for these lavish picnics. Imagine the Snacking Socialites sipping vintage wines beneath the shade of the historic Central Park

Conservatory Garden, where the beauty of the blooms is as captivating as the culinary creations.

- **Landmarks and Luxuries**: As we savor these moments of "Picnic Perfection," we'll intertwine our journey with Manhattan's iconic landmarks. Picture enjoying a gourmet picnic at Strawberry Fields, paying tribute to John Lennon's legacy, or indulging in a Central Park brunch with skyline views of the renowned Dakota building.

- **Artisanal Cheese Selection**: Immerse yourself in the world of artisanal cheeses as the Snacking Socialites curate cheese platters that are a testament to Manhattan's gourmet culture. Imagine sampling aged Gouda, creamy Camembert, and blue-veined Roquefort, all paired with honeycomb and artisanal crackers at a picturesque spot near Central Park's Conservatory Water.

- **Champagne and Caviar Indulgence**: Join us for a champagne and caviar extravaganza amidst Central Park's beauty, where the Snacking Socialites elevate picnicking to new heights. Picture sipping on vintage champagne while savoring delicate caviar-topped blinis near the iconic Alice in Wonderland sculpture, creating an unforgettable gourmet experience.

- **Lakeside Dining**: Explore the charm of lakeside picnics, where the Snacking Socialites gather by the tranquil waters of Central Park's Jacqueline Kennedy Onassis Reservoir.

In Manhattan, darling, even a picnic becomes an opportunity to make a statement, showcasing your style, substance, and flair for spontaneity. These picnics reflect the city's dedication to sophistication and the celebration of life against the backdrop of its iconic landmarks. Stay tuned, dear readers, as we continue to explore the world of "Picnic Perfection" amidst the grandeur of Gotham, where every bite and every view is a testament to the city's timeless allure and the remarkable stories it continues to tell.

Completed Tasks: Picnic Perfection Activities

Action Items: Intentions and Thoughts

EAT LIKE AN A-LISTER

Elevated Outdoor Eats

In the enchanting realm of Manhattan's Central Park, where the city's vibrant pulse harmonizes with nature's serenity, there exists a culinary movement known as "Elevated Outdoor Eats." These al fresco dining experiences are not mere picnics; they are gastronomic journeys that rival the finest restaurants, all set against the backdrop of the city's most iconic landmarks. Join me, darlings, as we delve into the world of "Elevated Outdoor Eats," where every bite is a celebration of style, substance, and sophistication, intertwined with the landmarks that define the Manhattan landscape.

➢ **Champagne and Lobster Extravaganza**: Explore the world of champagne and lobster extravaganzas, where the Snacking Socialites sip on vintage bubbles and indulge in succulent lobster dishes amidst the lush beauty of Central Park's Conservatory Garden. Picture a gourmet picnic that pays homage to the city's rich history and culinary culture.

➢ **Skyline Soirées**: Immerse yourself in the charm of rooftop soirées within Central Park, where every outdoor dining experience offers panoramic views of the Manhattan skyline. Imagine savoring dishes like truffle-infused foie gras and decadent chocolate desserts, all while lounging beneath the stars and the shadow of the iconic San Remo building.

➢ **Wine Tasting with a View**: Join us for wine tasting experiences that blend the art of viticulture with the beauty of Central Park's natural landscapes. Picture the Snacking Socialites sipping on rare vintages while overlooking the Jacqueline Kennedy Onassis Reservoir, creating a fusion of flavor and serenity.

➢ **Iconic Picnic Settings**: Delve into the magic of picnics set against Central Park's iconic landmarks, where every bite becomes a moment of cultural appreciation. Imagine enjoying a Central Park brunch with skyline views near the famed Bethesda Terrace or indulging in a Shakespearean-inspired picnic near the Delacorte Theater, where the Bard's classics come to life.

➤ **Sushi Under the Stars**: Immerse yourself in the world of rooftop sushi soirées, where the Snacking Socialites indulge in the art of sushi beneath the Manhattan night sky. Picture savoring exquisite nigiri and sashimi creations while gazing at the sparkling lights of the Empire State Building and the Chrysler Building.

➤ **Secret Garden Feasts**: Explore the charm of secret garden feasts amidst Central Park's hidden alcoves and serene corners. Join us as the Snacking Socialites transform these tranquil spots into gourmet dining stages, complete with decadent dishes and fine wines that celebrate the beauty of nature.

➤ **Theatrical Picnics**: Delve into the world of theatrical picnics, where the Snacking Socialites combine their love for the arts with culinary delights. Imagine attending Shakespearean picnics near the Delacorte Theater, where each dish is inspired by the classics and enjoyed as part of a cultural experience.

➤ **Chocolate and Central Park**: Join us for chocolate-themed picnics that are a delightful blend of indulgence and natural beauty. Picture savoring gourmet chocolates, truffles, and cocoa-infused treats while surrounded by the lush greenery of Central Park's Great Lawn.

In the world of "Elevated Outdoor Eats," every outdoor dining experience is a work of culinary art, a celebration of style, and a nod to Manhattan's enduring glamour. Stay tuned, dear readers, as we continue to uncover the secrets of creating unforgettable al fresco dining moments amidst the grandeur of Central Park, where every bite and every view is a testament to the city's ability to combine sophistication and spontaneity, creating dining experiences as legendary as the city itself.

Completed Tasks: Outdoor Eats Activities

Inspirational Quote

GOOD, BETTER, BEST. NEVER LET IT REST. 'TIL YOUR GOOD IS BETTER
AND YOUR BETTER IS BEST.' — St. Jerome

Action Items: Intentions and Thoughts

The Charms of Central Park

In the enchanting heart of Manhattan, where the city's energy finds solace in nature's embrace, Central Park reigns as an iconic oasis of tranquility. Amidst its hidden alcoves, sunlit glades, and serene ponds lies a world of al fresco dining, where the culinary movement known as "The Charms of Central Park" takes center stage. These picnics are not just about savoring gourmet delights; they are love letters to the park's beauty and Manhattan's landmarks. Join me, darlings, as we explore "The Charms of Central Park," where every bite is a serenade to style, substance, and the city's timeless allure, intertwined with the iconic landmarks that define the Manhattan landscape.

➢ **Botanical Picnic Bliss**: Immerse yourself in the enchanting world of botanical picnics, where Central Park's gardens serve as the backdrop for themed feasts. Picture a cherry blossom picnic in the Conservatory Garden, complete with sushi rolls inspired by Japanese Hanami traditions and floral-infused cocktails, all amidst the blooms and beauty of the garden.

➢ **Lakeside Dining**: Explore the allure of lakeside picnics, where the Snacking Socialites gather by the tranquil waters of Central Park's Jacqueline Kennedy Onassis Reservoir. Imagine indulging in a Mediterranean-inspired picnic with mezze platters and sangria, all while gazing at the picturesque Manhattan skyline reflected in the water.

➢ **Secret Garden Feasts**: Delve into the charm of secret garden feasts, where the Snacking Socialites transform hidden alcoves and serene corners into gourmet dining stages. Picture enjoying an intimate picnic in the Shakespeare Garden, where Shakespearean sonnets set the mood, and each dish is an ode to the classics.

➢ **Landmarks and Luxuries**: As we savor "The Charms of Central Park," we'll intertwine our journey with Manhattan's iconic landmarks. Imagine enjoying a gourmet picnic near the iconic Bow Bridge, where the skyline creates a breathtaking backdrop, or savoring a Central Park brunch near the Bethesda Terrace, where the grandeur of the location matches the culinary excellence.

➤ **Autumn Picnic Splendor**: Immerse yourself in the splendor of autumn picnics, where the Snacking Socialites celebrate Central Park's changing colors. Picture savoring seasonal delights like pumpkin bisque and caramel apple tartlets amidst a tapestry of vibrant foliage near the iconic Gapstow Bridge.

➤ **Bike Picnic Adventures**: Explore the world of bike picnics, where the Snacking Socialites combine leisurely rides through Central Park with gourmet feasts. Imagine pedaling to idyllic spots like The Mall and Literary Walk for a brunch picnic complete with artisanal pastries and freshly squeezed juices.

➤ **Musical Picnics**: Delve into the magic of musical picnics, where the Snacking Socialites enjoy live performances in Central Park's concert venues. Picture dining al fresco before a night of enchanting music at the Naumburg Bandshell, where every note becomes a part of the dining experience.

In Manhattan, dear readers, even a picnic becomes an opportunity to celebrate the city's timeless allure, showcasing elegance, eclecticism, and a touch of the unexpected. These "Charms of Central Park" reflect the city's commitment to sophistication and the celebration of life against the backdrop of its most treasured landmarks. Stay tuned as we continue to explore the world of al fresco dining amidst the grandeur of Gotham, where every bite and every vista is a testament to the remarkable stories that Manhattan continues to tell.

EAT LIKE AN A-LISTER

Completed Tasks: Central Park Charm Activities

Action Items: Intentions and Thoughts

EAT LIKE AN A-LISTER

Nature's Serenade

In the heart of Manhattan, where the city's relentless pulse finds harmony in the serenity of Central Park, a culinary movement known as "Nature's Serenade" takes center stage. These al fresco dining experiences are not just picnics; they are symphonies of style, substance, and spontaneity, set against the backdrop of the city's most iconic landmarks. Join me, darlings, as we explore "Nature's Serenade," where every bite is a celebration of nature's beauty, intertwined with the iconic landmarks that define the Manhattan landscape.

> ➢ **Picnicking by the Reservoir**: Delve into the magic of picnics by the tranquil waters of Central Park's Jacqueline Kennedy Onassis Reservoir. Imagine indulging in a Mediterranean-inspired feast with mezze platters and sangria, all while gazing at the picturesque Manhattan skyline mirrored in the water.

> ➢ **Twilight Elegance**: Explore the allure of twilight picnics, where the Snacking Socialites revel in the enchantment of Central Park at sundown. Picture a candlelit dinner near the iconic Bethesda Terrace, where the city's lights begin to twinkle, creating an atmosphere that's pure Manhattan magic.

> ➢ **Champagne and Stargazing**: Immerse yourself in the world of champagne and stargazing picnics, where the Snacking Socialites sip on bubbly while lying on blankets beneath the vast night sky. Imagine toasting to the stars near the Great Lawn, where the constellations become part of the dining experience.

> ➢ **Musical Al Fresco**: Delve into the magic of musical al fresco dining, where the Snacking Socialites enjoy live performances amidst Central Park's natural beauty. Picture savoring a gourmet picnic before a night of enchanting music at the iconic Delacorte Theater, where the Bard's classics come to life.

➢ **Autumnal Euphoria**: Immerse yourself in the enchantment of autumnal picnics, where the Snacking Socialites celebrate Central Park's foliage in its fiery glory. Picture savoring seasonal delights like butternut squash soup and spiced apple tarts amidst a tapestry of vibrant fall colors near the iconic Conservatory Garden.

➢ **Moonlit Bike Picnics**: Explore the world of moonlit bike picnics, where the Snacking Socialites combine nighttime rides through Central Park with gourmet feasts. Imagine pedaling to secluded spots like Shakespeare Garden for a midnight picnic with champagne and exquisite desserts.

➢ **Theatrical Twilight**: Delve into the world of theatrical twilight picnics, where the Snacking Socialites dine al fresco before attending performances in Central Park's historic theaters. Picture enjoying a candlelit dinner near the Delacorte Theater, where Shakespearean classics come to life under the starry sky.

➢ **Starry Skies and Skyline Views**: Join us for picnics under the starry skies, where the Snacking Socialites indulge in gourmet delights while taking in Manhattan's iconic skyline views. Imagine dining with the city's lights as a backdrop near the picturesque Bow Bridge, creating an ambiance that's pure Manhattan magic.

In Manhattan, dear readers, even a picnic becomes an opportunity to celebrate the city's timeless allure, showcasing elegance, eclecticism, and a dash of the unexpected. These moments of "Nature's Serenade" reflect the city's commitment to sophistication and the celebration of life amidst its most treasured landmarks. Stay tuned as we continue to explore the world of al fresco dining amidst the grandeur of Gotham, where every bite and every vista is a testament to the remarkable stories that Manhattan continues to tell.

EAT LIKE AN A-LISTER

Completed Tasks: Nature's Serenade Activities

Inspirational Quote

I LEARNED THAT WE CAN DO ANYTHING, BUT WE CAN'T DO EVERYTHING . . . AT LEAST NOT AT THE SAME TIME. SO, THINK OF YOUR PRIORITIES NOT IN TERMS OF WHAT ACTIVITIES YOU DO, BUT WHEN YOU DO THEM. TIMING IS EVERYTHING. — Dan Millman

70

Action Items: Intentions and Thoughts

Action Items: Intentions and Thoughts

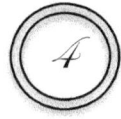

4

Broadway Bites:
Power Breakfasts to Kickstart Your Day

Manhattan—a city that awakens not with the chirping of birds but with the fervent aspirations of its inhabitants, each dawn whispering tales of ambition and the audacious hope of making it big. Here, mornings aren't just the start of a new day; they are a grand overture to the day's forthcoming drama. And what better way to take on the city's rhythm than with a breakfast that's as robust and rousing as Broadway's opening number?

Envision this: You're seated at a chic bistro just off Times Square, and as the city's pulse quickens outside, every eye inside is irresistibly drawn to you. Not because of the brand of your shoes, but the dynamism with which you command your morning feast. Honey, that's the Broadway Breakfast Bravura—a performance in itself, blending sustenance with showmanship.

In this enticing chapter of The Manhattan Diaries, we dive deep into the world of energizing eats. From the velvety smoothies that echo melodies of distant tropical lands to the avant-garde avocado toasts that resonate with innovation, you'll master the art of a breakfast that's both nourishing and noteworthy.

But, it's not just about the flavors. It's the mindset. It's about gearing up for your role in the grand play that is Manhattan. About intertwining nutrition with narrative, starting your day with a prologue that promises both purpose and panache.

So, accompany me as we sashay through the famed streets, tasting the morning offerings that empower the city's movers and shakers. Because, darling, in Manhattan, every breakfast is a prelude to potential greatness. Ready yourself, take that first invigorating sip of your espresso, and set the scene. Welcome to The Manhattan Diaries—where your morning can be as dazzling as the neon lights of Broadway.

Rise and Shine Smoothies

In the whirlwind of Manhattan's mornings, where ambition meets the relentless pace of the city, "Rise and Shine Smoothies" emerge as the secret elixirs of success. Picture this, darlings: You're at a trendy juice bar in the heart of Midtown Manhattan, and as the city awakens outside, your choice of morning elixir becomes an artful statement of vigor and vitality. These smoothies are not mere beverages; they are the orchestrations of a vibrant city's heartbeat, promising to infuse your day with the energy it demands. Dive into the world of "Rise and Shine Smoothies," where each sip is a serenade to Manhattan's grandeur and an ode to the landmarks that define it.

➢ **Sunrise Citrus Burst**: Start your day with a burst of citrusy goodness, a blend of fresh oranges, grapefruits, and a hint of lemon, reminiscent of the sun rising over the East River. Imagine sipping this zesty concoction near the iconic Brooklyn Bridge, where the skyline unfolds before your eyes.

➢ **Berry Bliss Awakening**: Indulge in a berry-packed smoothie that awakens your senses with a symphony of strawberries, blueberries, and raspberries. Picture savoring this vibrant blend near the bustling Times Square, where the city's energy matches the vibrancy of your breakfast.

➢ **Manhattan Green Vitality**: Embrace the urban vitality with a Manhattan Green smoothie, blending kale, spinach, and avocado for a nutrient-packed start to your day. Imagine enjoying this green elixir near Central Park, where nature's beauty and city's hustle converge in harmony.

➢ **Broadway Banana Delight**: Delight in a Broadway-inspired banana smoothie that combines the sweetness of ripe bananas with a touch of Broadway magic—vanilla and cinnamon. Picture sipping this delectable treat near the iconic Radio City Music Hall, where the city's entertainment legacy is celebrated.

➤ **Tropical Morning Escape**: Transport yourself to a tropical paradise with a pineapple-infused smoothie that combines pineapple, coconut, and a splash of passionfruit. Imagine sipping this exotic blend near the iconic Statue of Liberty, where Lady Liberty welcomes you with open arms.

➤ **Empire State Elixir**: Embrace the boldness of the city with an Empire State Elixir that boasts a mix of coffee, chocolate, and a dash of New York-style confidence. Picture enjoying this coffee-infused delight near the Empire State Building, where the city's skyline is a testament to ambition.

➤ **Mango Manhattan Mingle**: Dive into the sweet embrace of a Mango Manhattan Mingle, a smoothie that blends ripe mangoes with a hint of mint for a refreshing kick. Imagine savoring this tropical treat near the historic Flatiron Building, where old-world charm meets modern Manhattan.

➤ **Mango Manhattan Mingle**: Dive into the sweet embrace of a Mango Manhattan Mingle, a smoothie that blends ripe mangoes with a hint of mint for a refreshing kick. Imagine savoring this tropical treat near the historic Flatiron Building, where old-world charm meets modern Manhattan.

In the world of "Rise and Shine Smoothies," every sip is a journey through Manhattan's diverse landscapes, and each flavor is an ode to the city's vibrant spirit. Stay tuned, dear readers, as we continue to uncover the secrets of starting your Manhattan mornings with the vigor and vitality they deserve, all while embracing the grandeur of the city and the landmarks that make it legendary.

Completed Tasks: Morning Smoothies Activities

_____

_____

_____

_____

_____

_____

_____

_____

_____

_____

_____

_____

_____

_____

_____

_____

_____

_____

_____

_____

_____

_____

_____

_____

_____

_____

Inspirational Quote

LIFE IS A LOT LIKE JAZZ . . . IT'S BEST WHEN YOU IMPROVISE. — George Gershwin

Action Items: Intentions and Thoughts

Avocado Toast: The New York Way

In the heart of Manhattan's bustling breakfast scene, where ambition meets innovation, "Avocado Toast: The New York Way" emerges as the quintessential morning indulgence. Picture this, darlings: You're at a chic cafe in the trendy Meatpacking District, and your plate of avocado toast isn't just a meal; it's an avant-garde masterpiece that redefines breakfast classics. These toasts aren't mere dishes; they are statements of culinary flair and New York-style audacity. Join me as we dive into the world of "Avocado Toast: The New York Way," where each bite is a celebration of Manhattan's dynamic spirit and an homage to the landmarks that define it.

- ➤ **Metropolitan Classic**: Savor the timeless elegance of a Metropolitan Classic avocado toast, featuring perfectly ripe avocados, heirloom tomatoes, and a drizzle of extra-virgin olive oil. Imagine indulging in this classic interpretation near the historic Brownstones of Brooklyn Heights, where old-world charm meets modern allure.

- ➤ **Spicy SoHo Surprise**: Embark on a culinary adventure with the Spicy SoHo Surprise avocado toast, a fusion of creamy avocados, fiery jalapeños, and a sprinkle of chili flakes. Picture relishing this bold creation near the vibrant streets of SoHo, where the city's artistic soul is on full display.

- ➤ **Midtown Manhattan Delight**: Elevate your morning with the Midtown Manhattan Delight avocado toast, adorned with poached eggs, truffle oil, and a sprinkle of microgreens. Imagine enjoying this indulgent masterpiece near the iconic Grand Central Terminal, where Manhattan's history converges with contemporary elegance.

- ➤ **Central Park Brunch Bliss**: Embrace the tranquility of a Central Park Brunch Bliss avocado toast, featuring avocado, smoked salmon, and a drizzle of lemon-infused olive oil. Picture savoring this brunch delight near the scenic Bethesda Terrace, where nature and sophistication coexist.

➢ **Greenwich Village Fusion**: Immerse yourself in the artistic spirit of Greenwich Village with a fusion avocado toast that combines creamy avocados with sun-dried tomatoes and balsamic glaze. Imagine savoring this artistic creation near Washington Square Park, where creativity flows like the nearby fountain.

➢ **Brooklyn Brunch Elegance**: Embrace Brooklyn's charm with a Brooklyn Brunch Elegance avocado toast adorned with avocado, goat cheese, honey, and crushed pistachios. Picture enjoying this exquisite delight near the iconic DUMBO waterfront, where the Manhattan Bridge frames your view.

➢ **Chinatown Spice**: Embark on a culinary adventure with a Chinatown Spice avocado toast, featuring avocados, pickled ginger, and a dash of soy sauce. Imagine savoring this bold creation near the vibrant streets of Chinatown, where the city's flavors come alive.

➢ **Chelsea Market Indulgence**: Delight in the Chelsea Market Indulgence avocado toast, topped with creamy avocado, burrata cheese, and a drizzle of balsamic reduction. Picture indulging in this culinary masterpiece near the bustling Chelsea Market, where gourmet delights await at every corner.

In the world of "Avocado Toast: The New York Way," every bite is a journey through Manhattan's diverse culinary landscape, and each flavor is an homage to the city's dynamic spirit. Stay tuned, dear readers, as we continue to uncover the secrets of savoring Manhattan mornings with culinary audacity, all while embracing the grandeur of the city and the landmarks that make it legendary.

Completed Tasks: Avocado Toast Activities

_____

_____

_____

_____

_____

_____

_____

_____

_____

_____

_____

_____

_____

_____

_____

_____

_____

_____

_____

_____

_____

_____

_____

_____

_____

_____

_____

_____

Inspirational Quote

IT'S NOT ABOUT HIDING YOUR IMPERFECTIONS ON A SHOOT; IT'S ABOUT EMBRACING THEM AND BEING UNAPOLOGETIC ABOUT THEM. — Erin O'Connor

BROADWAY BITES

Action Items: Intentions and Thoughts

EAT LIKE AN A-LISTER

Breakfast with a View

In the vivacious world of Manhattan mornings, where every day unfolds like a new chapter in the city's grand narrative, "Breakfast with a View" takes center stage. Picture this, darlings: You're perched at an elegant rooftop restaurant, and as the sun bathes the city in golden light, your breakfast becomes a masterpiece set against the backdrop of Manhattan's iconic landmarks. These breakfasts aren't mere meals; they are symphonies of flavor and aesthetics, where nourishment meets breathtaking vistas. Join me as we embark on a journey into the realm of "Breakfast with a View," where each bite is a celebration of Manhattan's grandeur and an homage to the landmarks that define it.

- ➢ **Sunrise Over the Skyline**: Savor the enchantment of a Sunrise over the Skyline breakfast, featuring fresh pastries, gourmet coffee, and panoramic views of the Manhattan skyline. Imagine indulging in this morning feast near the elegant Empire State Building, where the city's ambitions touch the sky.

- ➢ **Lady Liberty Brunch**: Embrace the liberty of flavors with a Lady Liberty Brunch that pairs decadent French toast with mimosas, all while gazing at the Statue of Liberty in the distance. Picture relishing this indulgent treat near Battery Park, where history and modernity converge.

- ➢ **Central Park Serenity**: Immerse yourself in the serenity of a Central Park Serenity breakfast, featuring seasonal fruits, artisanal cheeses, and the gentle rustle of leaves. Imagine savoring this idyllic feast near the iconic Bow Bridge, where the city's hustle and bustle give way to nature's embrace.

- ➢ **Highline Delights**: Delight in the flavors of the Highline with a breakfast that combines fresh berries, Greek yogurt, and honey, all while overlooking the elevated High Line Park. Picture enjoying this wholesome treat near the Chelsea Market, where the city's diversity thrives.

➢ **Brooklyn Bridge Breakfast**: Start your day with a Brooklyn Bridge Breakfast, featuring freshly baked bagels, lox, and cream cheese, all while taking in the majestic view of the Brooklyn Bridge. Imagine savoring this New York classic near the historic bridge's promenade, where history meets modern elegance.

➢ **Skyscraper Sunrise**: Embrace the dawn with a Skyscraper Sunrise breakfast that offers a medley of seasonal fruits, granola, and a skyline view that stretches as far as the eye can see. Picture enjoying this healthy and invigorating meal near the Top of the Rock Observation Deck, where the city's grandeur unfolds beneath you.

➢ **Museum Mile Morning**: Immerse yourself in culture and cuisine with a Museum Mile morning breakfast, combining a continental spread with a view of the world-famous Museum Mile. Imagine indulging in this artistic feast near the steps of The Metropolitan Museum of Art, where art and breakfast become a harmonious experience.

➢ **City that Never Sleeps**: Dive into the vibrant energy of a City that Never Sleeps breakfast, featuring New York-style bagels, a variety of spreads, and a view of the bustling city streets below. Picture relishing this quintessential Manhattan breakfast near Times Square, where the city's lights shine day and night.

In the world of "Breakfast with a View," every bite is a journey through Manhattan's diverse culinary landscape, and each view is a testament to the city's timeless allure. Stay tuned, dear readers, as we continue to uncover the secrets of savoring Manhattan mornings with grandeur and elegance, all while embracing the city's iconic landmarks that make each breakfast an unforgettable experience.

EAT LIKE AN A-LISTER

Completed Tasks: Breakfast with a View Activities

Inspirational Quote

I DON'T LISTEN TO WHAT PEOPLE SAY ABOUT ME, AND I DON'T READ WHAT THEY WRITE ABOUT ME. PEOPLE CAN COMPARE ME TO ANYONE THEY WANT TO, BUT I'M NOT GOING TO WORRY ABOUT IT. —— Eric Davis

84

BROADWAY BITES

Action Items: Intentions and Thoughts

EAT LIKE AN A-LISTER

Mindset and Morning Rituals

In the heart of Manhattan's dynamic mornings, where ambition meets aspiration, "Mindset and Morning Rituals" take center stage. Picture this, darlings: You're at the dawn of a new day, surrounded by the city's iconic landmarks, and your morning rituals become a symphony of intention and inspiration. These rituals aren't just habits; they are the secret sauce of Manhattan's high achievers, blending motivation with Manhattan's unmistakable charisma. Join me as we embark on a journey into the realm of "Mindset and Morning Rituals," where each practice is a celebration of Manhattan's grandeur and an homage to the landmarks that define it.

> ➤ **Zen in the Financial District**: Start your day with Zen in the Financial District, where Wall Street's bustling energy meets morning meditation. Imagine finding your center amidst the Financial District's iconic skyscrapers, where ambition and serenity coexist.

> ➤ **Literary Mornings in Harlem**: Embrace the power of literature with Literary Mornings in Harlem, where reading and reflection become the cornerstone of your day. Picture immersing yourself in a classic novel at the Schomburg Center for Research in Black Culture, where Harlem's literary legacy thrives.

> ➤ **Fitness by the Brooklyn Bridge**: Energize your morning with Fitness by the Brooklyn Bridge, where a workout routine blends seamlessly with breathtaking views. Imagine jogging along the Brooklyn Bridge promenade, where the bridge's historic charm motivates your every step.

> ➤ **Culinary Creativity in Chelsea**: Unleash your culinary creativity with a morning cooking class in Chelsea, where art meets gastronomy. Picture experimenting with gourmet dishes at the

Institute of Culinary Education, just a stone's throw away from Chelsea Market's culinary delights.

➤ **Harmonious Harlem Jazz**: Kickstart your day with the Harmonious Harlem Jazz ritual, where you immerse yourself in the soulful melodies of Harlem's historic jazz clubs. Imagine letting the music set the tone for your morning near the legendary Apollo Theater, where musical legends have graced the stage.

➤ **Riverside Morning Ride**: Infuse your morning with energy through the Riverside Morning Ride, a cycling adventure along the scenic Hudson River Greenway. Picture pedaling with the city's skyline as your backdrop, near the vibrant Riverside Park, where nature and urban life converge.

➤ **Sunrise Yoga in Battery Park**: Find inner peace with Sunrise Yoga in Battery Park, a serene practice overlooking the Statue of Liberty and the harbor. Imagine greeting the day with sun salutations and gentle breezes near the Battery Park Esplanade, where tranquility reigns.

➤ **Morning Pages at the New York Public Library**: Ignite your creativity with Morning Pages at the New York Public Library, where you dedicate the early hours to journaling and self-reflection.

In the world of "Mindset and Morning Rituals," every practice is a journey through Manhattan's diverse landscapes, and each moment is an opportunity to harness the city's boundless energy. Stay tuned, dear readers, as we continue to uncover the secrets of embracing the morning with intention and inspiration, all while embracing the grandeur of the city and the landmarks that make each ritual a transformative experience. In Manhattan, every morning is a canvas to paint your aspirations, and every landmark is a reminder of the city's enduring spirit.

Completed Tasks: Mindset Morning Rituals Activities

_____

_____

_____

_____

_____

_____

_____

_____

_____

_____

_____

_____

_____

_____

_____

_____

_____

_____

_____

_____

_____

_____

_____

_____

_____

_____

_____

Inspirational Quote

THE WRIGHT BROTHERS FLEW RIGHT THROUGH THE SMOKE SCREEN OF IMPOSSIBILITY. — Charles Kettering

Action Items: Intentions and Thoughts

Action Items: Intentions and Thoughts

Fifth Avenue Feasts: Dinners Worthy of the Front Row at Fashion Week

Manhattan—a city where elegance is not just an accessory; it's an attitude. A place where each dusk doesn't signal an end but the onset of an enchanting nocturnal ballet. Amidst the twilight hues, the city doesn't just dine—it celebrates, each meal echoing tales of opulence, desire, and an undeniable taste for the exquisite. To dine in Manhattan isn't merely about sating hunger; it's about devouring the very essence of style and sophistication.

Picture this: You're gracefully descending the steps of a grand eatery on Fifth Avenue, each glance sent your way not captivated by the sequins of your gown, but by the elegance with which you carry your appetite. That, my dear, is the Fifth Avenue Food Flair, an epicurean escapade that's as revered as the front row at Fashion Week—a place where culinary craft meets couture.

In this tantalizing chapter of The Manhattan Diaries, we'll dive into the gourmet galaxies of the city's elite dining. From the tantalizing truffles that flirt with your palate to the champagne that dances effervescently with your aspirations, you'll uncover the art of dining with discernment and dazzle.

Yet, this journey isn't solely about the palate. It's a symphony of senses. It's about absorbing the ambiance, relishing the rhythm of sparkling conversations, and savoring every morsel as if it tells a tale. It's about recognizing that amidst the towering skyscrapers, there exists an equally towering legacy of culinary brilliance.

So, let's embark on this delectable journey, sampling bites that have witnessed countless deals and dreams. Because, darling, in Manhattan, every dinner is not just a meal—it's a statement, a narrative, an art form. Ready your forks and your finest frocks; the city's dining stage beckons. Welcome to The Manhattan Diaries—where your dinner can be as dazzling as the Fifth Avenue's glittering facades.

Champagne Soirees: Sipping Elegance on the Golden Mile

In the dazzling world of Manhattan's high society, where elegance is nonnegotiable and sophistication is a way of life, "Champagne Soirees: Sipping Elegance on the Golden Mile" takes center stage. Picture this, darlings: You're perched at an exclusive venue along the illustrious Fifth Avenue, the sparkling city skyline as your backdrop, and a flute of the finest champagne in your hand. These champagne soirees aren't just gatherings; they are symphonies of opulence and style. Join me as we embark on a journey into the realm of "Champagne Soirees," where each sip is a celebration of Manhattan's grandeur and an homage to the landmarks that define it.

➢ **The Plaza Pinnacle**: Immerse yourself in the timeless elegance of The Plaza Hotel, where champagne flows like a river of liquid gold. Imagine indulging in effervescent luxury near Central Park, where the city's green heart meets high society.

➢ **Metropolitan Magic**: Experience the enchantment of the Metropolitan Museum of Art's rooftop garden, where art and champagne unite in perfect harmony. Picture yourself sipping bubbly amidst the beauty of the museum's exquisite rooftop, overlooking the iconic skyline.

➢ **Gotham Glamour at Tiffany's**: Step into the world of Audrey Hepburn with a champagne soirée at Tiffany & Co.'s flagship store on Fifth Avenue. Imagine toasting to your heart's desires near the legendary Tiffany's windows, where dreams of elegance come to life.

➢ **The Gilded Garden at St. Regis**: Revel in the lavishness of the St. Regis Hotel's King Cole Bar, where champagne is served in an atmosphere of timeless sophistication. Picture yourself savoring bubbly in a setting that echoes the grandeur of the Gilded Age, near the historic King Cole mural.

- ➤ **Sundown Splendor at The Peninsula**: Bask in the golden hour's glow with a champagne soirée at The Peninsula New York's rooftop terrace. Imagine sipping champagne as the sun sets behind the iconic Peninsula clock, where luxury meets the skyline.

- ➤ **MoMA Magic**: Elevate your evening with a champagne gathering at The Museum of Modern Art's Sculpture Garden. Picture yourself surrounded by world-class art, sipping bubbly in an oasis of creativity amidst the city's cultural landmarks.

- ➤ **Sunset Serenity at The High Line**: Experience the tranquility of a champagne soirée along the High Line's elevated park, where urban oasis meets artful elegance. Imagine toasting to the Manhattan skyline's changing colors as the day turns into night.

- ➤ **Gatsby-Inspired Glamour**: Transport yourself to the Roaring Twenties with a Gatsby-inspired champagne soirée at a hidden speakeasy along Fifth Avenue. Picture yourself sipping champagne in an intimate setting reminiscent of Fitzgerald's era, where secrets and sophistication reign.

In the world of "Champagne Soirees," every sip is a journey through Manhattan's glamorous nightlife, and each venue is a testament to the city's timeless allure. Stay tuned, dear readers, as we continue to uncover the secrets of sipping elegance on the Golden Mile, all while embracing the grandeur of the city and the landmarks that make each soirée a sparkling memory. In Manhattan, every champagne flute is a symbol of style, and every landmark is a reminder of the city's enduring charm. Cheers to the Manhattan Diaries' champagne-soaked elegance!

Completed Tasks: Champagne Soirees Activities

Action Items: Intentions and Thoughts

Truffle Tales: A Culinary Romance with the Black Diamond

In the tantalizing world of Manhattan's haute cuisine, where every bite is a seduction and every dish a declaration of culinary sophistication, "Truffle Tales: A Culinary Romance with the Black Diamond" emerges as a delectable love story. Imagine, darlings, being ensconced in the lavish ambiance of a Michelin-starred restaurant along the city's bustling streets, the intoxicating aroma of truffles lingering in the air. These truffle tales aren't just meals; they are gastronomic affairs of the heart. Join me as we delve into the captivating realm of "Truffle Tales," where each bite is a celebration of Manhattan's grandeur and an homage to the landmarks that define it.

> ➤ **Per Se Poetry**: Embark on a culinary journey at Per Se, where each truffle-infused dish is a masterpiece. Imagine savoring the poetry of flavors near Columbus Circle, with Central Park as your backdrop.

> ➤ **Daniel's Epicurean Elegance**: Experience the epitome of culinary elegance at Restaurant Daniel, where truffles transform dishes into works of art. Picture yourself dining amid the Upper East Side's refined charm, near the esteemed Metropolitan Museum of Art.

> ➤ **Gramercy Truffle Delights**: Indulge in truffle delicacies at Gramercy Tavern, where rustic charm meets gourmet excellence. Imagine reveling in the warmth of Gramercy Park's neighborhood, where history and innovation intertwine.

> ➤ **NoMad's Truffle Tango**: Explore the culinary magic of The NoMad, where truffles add a touch of whimsy to each plate. Picture yourself in the vibrant NoMad district, where the building's history and culinary creativity collide.

> ➤ **L'Artusi's Truffle Temptations**: Immerse yourself in the culinary artistry of L'Artusi, where truffles enhance Italian-inspired dishes.

Picture dining in the heart of the West Village, where historic charm meets modern flair.

➢ **Elegant Evenings at Le Bernardin**: Embark on an elegant evening at Le Bernardin, where truffles elevate seafood to unparalleled heights. Imagine savoring exquisite flavors near the iconic sights of Midtown Manhattan.

➢ **Tavern on the Green's Truffle Treasures**: Delight in truffle treasures at Tavern on the Green, where the magic of Central Park meets gourmet extravagance. Picture a dining experience in the heart of the park, surrounded by nature's beauty.

➢ **Cosmopolitan Comfort at Ai Fiori**: Experience cosmopolitan comfort at Ai Fiori, where truffles add a touch of indulgence to classic dishes. Imagine dining in the heart of Midtown, where the city's energy is palpable.

➢ **Truffles at Eleven Madison Park's Pinnacle of Innovation**: Dive into the world of culinary innovation at Eleven Madison Park, where truffles are the stars of meticulously crafted dishes. Imagine dining with views of Madison Square Park, savoring flavors that reflect the spirit of Manhattan's avant-garde and the restaurant's iconic status

In the world of "Truffle Tales," each bite is a journey through Manhattan's gourmet landscape, and each restaurant is a testament to the city's culinary excellence. Stay tuned, dear readers, as we continue to explore the romance of truffles in the heart of Manhattan, all while embracing the grandeur of the city and the landmarks that make each truffle tale a savory memory. In Manhattan, every culinary creation is a symbol of style, and every landmark is a reminder of the city's timeless charm. Bon appétit to the Manhattan Diaries' truffle-infused romance!

Completed Tasks: Truffle Tales Activities

_____
_____
_____
_____
_____
_____
_____
_____
_____
_____
_____
_____
_____
_____
_____
_____
_____
_____
_____
_____
_____
_____
_____
_____
_____
_____

Inspirational Quote

LIFE IS TOO SHORT FOR LONG-TERM GRUDGES. — Elon Musk

Action Items: Intentions and Thoughts

Dining with the Stars: Celebrity Haunts Along the Golden Mile

In the glittering cosmos of Manhattan's high society, where fame, fortune, and fabulousness converge, "Dining with the Stars: Celebrity Haunts Along the Golden Mile" unfolds as a culinary escapade beyond compare. Picture this, darlings: You're seated at an exclusive restaurant along the iconic Fifth Avenue, the stylish cityscape serving as your backdrop, and a menu brimming with star-studded dishes. These celebrity haunts aren't just restaurants; they are theaters of glamour and gastronomy. Join me as we embark on a journey into the enchanting realm of "Dining with the Stars," where each meal is a celebration of Manhattan's grandeur and an homage to the landmarks that define it.

➢ **The Polo Bar**: Ralph Lauren's Equestrian Elegance: Dine in the presence of the fashion maestro's legacy, where equestrian-inspired decor meets impeccable American cuisine. Picture yourself indulging in Ralph Lauren's timeless vision amidst the chic Upper East Side.

➢ **The Grill**: A Culinary Revival at The Seagram Building: Savor classic American fare at The Grill, a beloved haunt of both celebrities and Manhattan's elite. Imagine dining in the historic Seagram Building, where Midtown's bustling energy meets Mid-Century Modern glamour.

➢ **The Rainbow Room**: Glamour at the Top of the Rock: Ascend to the iconic Rainbow Room, where timeless elegance meets breathtaking views. Picture yourself sipping cocktails and savoring gourmet delights while gazing at the city's skyline from Rockefeller Center.

➢ **Carbone's Red Sauce Romance**: Transport yourself to a bygone era at Carbone, where Italian-American cuisine and retro charm collide. Imagine dining in the heart of Greenwich Village, where the neighborhood's artistic spirit is palpable.

- **Nobu's Culinary Fusion**: Experience the fusion of Japanese and Peruvian flavors at Nobu Fifty Seven, a favorite of Hollywood's elite. Picture yourself dining amidst sleek design near Midtown's vibrant energy.

- **The Russian Tea Room's Artistic Opulence**: Dine in opulence at The Russian Tea Room, where Russian-inspired cuisine meets artistic decor. Imagine savoring indulgent dishes in a setting reminiscent of a Russian fairy tale near Carnegie Hall.

- **The Spotted Pig's Cozy Charm**: Revel in the cozy charm of The Spotted Pig, a gastropub known for its delectable British and Italian-inspired fare. Picture yourself enjoying comfort food in the heart of the West Village, where creativity and culinary excellence thrive.

- **Sant Ambroeus**: A Taste of Milan in Manhattan: Indulge in Milanese elegance at Sant Ambroeus, a haunt adored by fashion icons. Imagine sipping espresso and savoring Italian delicacies amidst the fashionable atmosphere of the Upper East Side.

- **Le Coucou's Parisian Elegance**: Step into a world of refined French dining at Le Coucou, a favorite among A-listers and culinary enthusiasts alike. Imagine savoring delicate French cuisine amidst elegant chandeliers and vintage decor in SoHo, where Manhattan's modern energy meets the romance of Paris.

In the world of "Dining with the Stars," each meal is a journey through Manhattan's culinary cosmos, and each restaurant is a testament to the city's cultural richness. Stay tuned, dear readers, as we continue to explore the allure of dining at celebrity-frequented establishments, all while embracing the grandeur of the city and the landmarks that make each dining experience a star-studded affair. In Manhattan, every culinary creation is a symbol of style, and every landmark is a reminder of the city's timeless allure. Bon appétit to the Manhattan Diaries' celebrity-filled gastronomy!

EAT LIKE AN A-LISTER

Completed Tasks: Celebrity Haunt Activities

Inspirational Quote

YOU'RE ALWAYS WITH YOURSELF, SO YOU MIGHT AS WELL ENJOY THE COMPANY. — Diane Von Furstenberg

Action Items: Intentions and Thoughts

Fashion Forward Feasts: Where Culinary Craft Meets Couture

In the dazzling world of Manhattan's haut monde, where style is paramount, and sophistication is non-negotiable, "Fashion Forward Feasts: Where Culinary Craft Meets Couture" emerges as an unparalleled culinary voyage. Envision this, darlings: You're seated at a chic eatery along the illustrious Fifth Avenue, where the fashion elite gather, and the menu is a runway of exquisite dishes. These fashion-forward feasts aren't just meals; they are expressions of haute cuisine, where culinary craft converges with couture. Join me as we embark on a journey into the glamorous realm of "Fashion Forward Feasts," where every bite is a celebration of Manhattan's grandeur and an homage to the landmarks that define it.

➢ **Boulud Sud's Mediterranean Chic**: Savor Mediterranean-inspired dishes at Boulud Sud, a haunt favored by the fashion crowd. Imagine dining amidst sleek design on the Upper West Side, where the city's artistic spirit is palpable.

➢ **Le Coucou: A Culinary Masterpiece in SoHo**: Delight in French-inspired fare at Le Coucou, where classic elegance meets contemporary charm. Picture yourself dining in the heart of SoHo, where artistic innovation and culinary excellence thrive.

➢ **The Modern's Artful Cuisine**: Experience artful cuisine at The Modern, a Michelin-starred gem at the Museum of Modern Art. Imagine savoring gourmet delights amidst the creativity of Midtown Manhattan.

➢ **Marea's Seafood Sensations**: Indulge in seafood sensations at Marea, where coastal Italian cuisine takes center stage. Picture yourself enjoying exquisite dishes near Central Park, where sophistication and natural beauty converge.

- ➢ **Ai Fiori's Italian Elegance**: Indulge in Italian elegance at Ai Fiori, where fine dining meets timeless style. Imagine savoring gourmet dishes in the heart of Midtown, where culinary excellence blends seamlessly with Manhattan's vibrant energy.

- ➢ **Gramercy Tavern's Artisanal Ambiance**: Dine amidst artisanal ambiance at Gramercy Tavern, a celebrated culinary gem. Picture yourself relishing farm-to-table cuisine in the charming Gramercy Park neighborhood, where authenticity and sophistication reign.

- ➢ **The Polo Bar**: Ralph Lauren's Culinary Couture: Experience Ralph Lauren's culinary couture at The Polo Bar, where American classics meet designer flair. Imagine dining amidst equestrian-inspired decor on the Upper East Side, where timeless style and gourmet creations harmonize.

- ➢ **ABC Kitchen's Sustainable Style**: Discover the fusion of sustainability and style at ABC Kitchen, where locally sourced ingredients meet a beautifully curated ambiance. Imagine dining in Union Square, surrounded by eco-chic decor that reflects Manhattan's commitment to both fashion and conscious dining.

In the world of "Fashion Forward Feasts," every meal is a journey through Manhattan's stylish culinary landscape, and each restaurant is a testament to the city's cultural richness. Stay tuned, dear readers, as we continue to explore the allure of dining at fashion-forward establishments, all while embracing the grandeur of the city and the landmarks that make each dining experience a fashionable affair. In Manhattan, every culinary creation is a symbol of sophistication, and every landmark is a reminder of the city's enduring allure. Bon appétit to the Manhattan Diaries' chic gastronomic adventures!

Completed Tasks: Fashion Forward Feasts Activities

_____

_____

_____

_____

_____

_____

_____

_____

_____

_____

_____

_____

_____

_____

_____

_____

_____

_____

_____

_____

_____

_____

_____

_____

_____

_____

_____

Inspirational Quote

THE IDEAL LIFE IS IN OUR BLOOD AND NEVER WILL BE STILL. — Phillips Brooks

Action Items: Intentions and Thoughts

Action Items: Intentions and Thoughts

6

SoHo Sips: Luxurious Liquids and Decadent Drinks for the Discerning Palate

Manhattan—a city that sips its secrets with a twinkle in its eye. Where every clink of crystal is not just a mere sound, but a toast to triumphs, dreams, and the audacity to dare. Here, in the heart of it all, where creativity and commerce intertwine, every drink isn't just about quenching thirst; it's about savoring the spirit of the city—with finesse, flair, and a touch of the fabulous.

Visualize: You're sauntering through the cobbled lanes of SoHo, eyes drawn to you, not because of the sparkle of your jewels, but the shimmer in your drink. That, darling, is the SoHo Sip Signature, a liquid allure that rivals even the most coveted couture, dripping with panache, flavor, and a touch of the unexpected.

In this intoxicating chapter of The Manhattan Diaries, we'll plunge into the world of Manhattan's most coveted cocktails and drinks. From the velvety vintage wines that whisper tales of bygone eras to the contemporary cocktails that fizz with the future, you'll learn the art of drinking with decadence and distinction.

But, it's more than just the taste. It's about the ambiance, the mood, the company. It's about immersing in the tales that each sip unravels, letting the liquid lace your soul with stories of Manhattan's luminaries. It's about reveling in both the limelight of the city's chic bars and the intimate shadows of its speakeasies, mastering the cocktail culture of Manhattan's core.

So, accompany me, as we swirl, sip, and savor the flavors echoing from SoHo's celebrated cellars and swanky spots. Because, sweetheart, in Manhattan, every sip is not just a drink—it's an experience, an embrace, a statement. Ready your senses for a journey of jubilant joy. Welcome to The Manhattan Diaries—where your drink can be as dramatic as the city's dazzling dreams.

The Art of Mixology at Employees Only

In the glittering tapestry of Manhattan's nightlife, where each evening is an invitation to revel in the city's unique rhythm, "The Art of Mixology at Employees Only" stands as a testament to craft, creativity, and cocktails that dance on the palate. Picture this, darlings: You're ensconced in the speakeasy allure of Employees Only, a gem of the West Village, where the art of mixology takes center stage. Here, each sip is a theatrical performance, and every cocktail is a masterpiece of taste and aesthetics. Join me as we delve into this intoxicating chapter of The Manhattan Diaries, where we'll explore the alchemy behind crafting the perfect cocktail, paying homage to the city's iconic landmarks that frame our spirited journey.

➤ **The Secrets of Speakeasies**: Unveil the secrets of speakeasies as we step into the hidden world of Employees Only, where clandestine allure meets inventive mixology.

➤ **The West Village Charisma**: Experience the charisma of the West Village, where historic charm and artistic energy create a backdrop for unforgettable evenings.

➤ **Cocktails as Art**: Delight in cocktails as a form of artistry, where the balance of flavors and presentation collide, evoking the spirit of Manhattan's creative heartbeat.

➤ **Greenwich Village's Timeless Appeal**: Immerse yourself in Greenwich Village's timeless appeal, where the neighborhood's history and bohemian spirit infuse every sip.

➤ **The Secrets of Speakeasies Unveiled**: Step into the world of speakeasies and uncover the intriguing secrets that lie within the doors of Employees Only. This hidden gem of the West Village encapsulates the clandestine allure of the Prohibition era, creating an ambiance where inventive mixology is the main act.

➢ **The Charisma of the West Village**: Immerse yourself in the irresistible charisma of the West Village, where historic cobblestone streets, artistic energy, and a vibrant nightlife converge to set the stage for unforgettable evenings. This neighborhood exudes an ageless charm that makes every visit an exploration of the city's timeless appeal.

➢ **Cocktails as Artistry**: Prepare to be delighted as you discover cocktails elevated to the status of art. At Employees Only, cocktails are not just beverages; they are masterpieces that combine the perfect balance of flavors, presentation, and innovation. Each sip is a sensory journey that encapsulates the creative heartbeat of Manhattan.

➢ **Greenwich Village's Timeless Enchantment**: Greenwich Village serves as the backdrop to this mixological adventure, and its timeless enchantment adds a unique dimension to the experience. With a rich history and a bohemian spirit, the Village infuses every cocktail with the essence of its eclectic character.

As we venture deeper into "The Art of Mixology at Employees Only," our exploration intertwines with Manhattan's iconic landmarks, where each cocktail becomes a sip of the city's diverse cultural tapestry. These libations are not mere drinks; they are expressions of Manhattan's ever-evolving creativity and the enchantment that permeates every corner of the city.

Stay tuned, dear readers, as we continue to uncover the irresistible allure of mixology at Employees Only, all while embracing the grandeur of the city and the landmarks that make each cocktail a tribute to Manhattan's enduring charm. In the city that never sleeps, every evening is a chance to raise a glass to life's pleasures, and every landmark is a reminder of its enduring allure. Cheers to The Manhattan Diaries' spirited mixology adventure!

Completed Tasks: The Art of Mixology Activities

Inspirational Quote

I LOVE THOSE WHO YEARN FOR THE IMPOSSIBLE. — Johann Wolfgang von Goethe

Action Items: Intentions and Thoughts

Craft Cocktails at Death and Co.

In the dazzling mosaic of Manhattan's nightlife, where each evening promises a rendezvous with the city's vivacious spirit, "Craft Cocktails at Death & Co." emerges as a masterpiece of libation artistry, style, and sophistication. Imagine this, my darlings: You're immersed in the intimate ambiance of Death & Co., a pioneer in the cocktail renaissance. Here, every sip is a voyage of taste, an exploration of creativity, and a toast to the city's timeless allure. Join me as we embark on this intoxicating chapter of The Manhattan Diaries, where we'll delve into the craft of cocktails, paying homage to the iconic landmarks that frame our spirited journey.

- ➤ **The Elegance of Death & Co.**: Step into the world of Death & Co., where elegance reigns supreme. This atmospheric haven in the East Village combines timeless charm with contemporary sophistication, creating a backdrop where craft cocktails take center stage.

- ➤ **East Village's Bohemian Energy**: Immerse yourself in the artistic energy of the East Village, where the neighborhood's bohemian spirit infuses every sip at Death & Co. With its historic roots and vibrant present, the East Village adds a unique charm to your mixology experience.

- ➤ **Crafting Cocktails as an Art Form**: At Death & Co., crafting cocktails is elevated to an art form. Each libation is a masterpiece, a harmonious blend of flavors and aesthetics that captivate both the senses and the soul. Every sip is an ode to innovation and tradition.

- ➤ **Manhattan's Cultural Heartbeat**: As you sip on your meticulously crafted cocktails at Death & Co., you'll be intertwined with Manhattan's cultural heartbeat. The city's landmarks, both historic and contemporary, serve as a backdrop to your mixological journey, reminding you that every cocktail is a sip of the city's dynamic narrative.

> **The Alchemical Ambiance**: Death & Co. immerses you in an alchemical ambiance, where the air is thick with creativity and anticipation. It's a place where cocktail craft is elevated to an art form, and every visit promises a journey of taste exploration.

> **East Village's Bohemian Canvas**: East Village's bohemian canvas sets the stage for your mixology adventure at Death & Co. With its eclectic history and vibrant present, this neighborhood infuses your libations with an extra layer of artistic charm, making each cocktail a work of liquid art.

> **Cocktail Culture Redefined**: At Death & Co., cocktail culture is not just about drinks; it's a lifestyle. With a commitment to precision and innovation, each libation is a testament to the endless possibilities of mixology. Every sip is a step into a world where tradition meets reinvention.

> Manhattan's Iconic Backdrop: While indulging in your craft cocktails at Death & Co., you'll be enveloped in Manhattan's iconic backdrop. The city's landmarks, whether historic theaters or modern skyscrapers, serve as a reminder that every cocktail tells a unique story in the grand narrative of Manhattan.

As we delve deeper into "Craft Cocktails at Death & Co.," we meld our exploration seamlessly with Manhattan's iconic landmarks, where each cocktail becomes a testament to the city's diverse cultural tapestry. These libations are not just drinks; they are expressions of Manhattan's unending creativity, where tradition and innovation converge.

EAT LIKE AN A-LISTER

Action Items: Intentions and Thoughts

Wine Adventures at La Compagnie des Vins Surnaturels

In the vibrant tapestry of Manhattan's culinary landscape, where every glass of wine tells a story, "Wine Adventures at La Compagnie des Vins Surnaturels" emerges as a haven for oenophiles seeking the extraordinary. Picture this, my darlings: You're ensconced in the enchanting ambiance of La Compagnie des Vins Surnaturels, a sanctuary in the heart of the city where each sip is a journey through the vineyards of the world. Join me as we uncork this captivating chapter of The Manhattan Diaries, delving into the art of wine, all while paying tribute to the iconic landmarks that frame our vinous exploration.

- ➤ **The Elegance of La Compagnie**: Step into the world of La Compagnie des Vins Surnaturels, where elegance reigns supreme. This sophisticated haven in NoHo combines timeless charm with an extensive wine selection, creating an atmosphere where wine takes center stage.

- ➤ **NoHo's Artistic Aura**: Immerse yourself in the artistic aura of NoHo, where creativity and culture converge. The neighborhood's historic roots and contemporary vibrancy add a unique charm to your wine adventure at La Compagnie, making every sip a fusion of art and taste.

- ➤ **A Wine Journey Beyond Borders**: At La Compagnie des Vins Surnaturels, the wine journey transcends borders. With a commitment to curating a diverse selection, each glass is a passport to a different terroir, a voyage that allows you to savor the essence of distant vineyards.

- ➤ **Manhattan's Cultural Kaleidoscope**: While you savor your meticulously chosen wines at La Compagnie, you'll be enveloped in Manhattan's cultural kaleidoscope. The city's iconic landmarks, both historic and contemporary, serve as a backdrop to your vinous adventure, reminding you that each wine tells a unique story in the grand narrative of Manhattan.

➤ **A Wine Connoisseur's Paradise**: La Compagnie des Vins Surnaturels is a haven for wine connoisseurs. Whether you're a seasoned aficionado or a budding enthusiast, the wine selection caters to a spectrum of tastes and knowledge levels. The knowledgeable sommeliers are at your service, guiding you through a vinous journey that promises discoveries and delights.

➤ **NoHo's Bohemian Reverie**: NoHo's bohemian reverie serves as the backdrop for your wine adventure. The neighborhood's eclectic mix of galleries, boutiques, and historic charm infuses every sip at La Compagnie with a touch of artistic allure. It's a place where creativity flows as freely as the wine.

➤ **Sipping History and Innovation**: At La Compagnie, you sip history and innovation in equal measure. Each wine is a testament to tradition, but also a showcase of modern winemaking excellence. It's a place where old-world classics harmonize with new-world innovations on your palate.

➤ **Manhattan's Iconic Canvas**: As you savor your chosen wines at La Compagnie, you're immersed in Manhattan's iconic canvas. The city's landmarks, whether the historic theaters of Broadway or the modern skyscrapers of Midtown, remind you that each wine is a brushstroke in the masterpiece that is Manhattan.

With every bottle uncorked at La Compagnie des Vins Surnaturels, we continue to intertwine our vinous exploration with the timeless landmarks of Manhattan. Each wine becomes a toast to the city's rich cultural tapestry, where diversity and sophistication converge.

Completed Tasks: Wine Adventures Activities

Inspirational Quote

EVERY MAN'S LIFE IS A FAIRYTALE WRITTEN BY GOD'S FINGERS. — Hans Christian Andersen

Action Items: Intentions and Thoughts

A Nightcap at The Roxy Hotel

In the enchanting chronicles of Manhattan's nightlife, where every night is a performance and every libation a serenade to the city's nocturnal allure, "A Nightcap at The Roxy Hotel" emerges as a quintessential chapter in the saga of sophistication and style. Imagine this, my darlings: You're ensconced in the timeless glamour of The Roxy Hotel, a sanctuary in the heart of TriBeCa where each sip is a melodious encore to your evening. Join me as we uncork this captivating chapter of The Manhattan Diaries, exploring the art of the nightcap, all while paying homage to the iconic landmarks that frame our nocturnal adventure.

➢ **The Roxy's Timeless Charm**: Step into the world of The Roxy Hotel, where timeless charm and contemporary cool coexist in harmony. This haven in TriBeCa offers a seductive ambiance that's equal parts vintage glamour and modern allure, creating the perfect setting for your nightcap.

➢ **TriBeCa's Artistic Aura**: Immerse yourself in the artistic aura of TriBeCa, where creativity thrives amidst cobblestone streets and historic warehouses. The neighborhood's eclectic blend of art, culture, and sophistication adds a unique flavor to your nightcap experience at The Roxy, making every sip a fusion of art and indulgence.

➢ **The Nightcap Symphony**: At The Roxy Hotel, the nightcap is more than a drink; it's a symphony of flavors and elegance. Each libation is crafted with precision, allowing you to savor the essence of the night while reveling in the rich notes of Manhattan's nocturnal spirit.

➢ **Manhattan's Timeless Night**: As you indulge in your chosen nightcap at The Roxy, you'll be enveloped in Manhattan's timeless night. The city's iconic landmarks, whether the historic streets of

TriBeCa or the shimmering lights of Lower Manhattan, serve as a backdrop to your nocturnal adventure, reminding you that every nightcap is a part of the city's enduring legacy.

> **Late-Night Jazz Serenades**: The Roxy Hotel is renowned for its late-night jazz serenades. Immerse yourself in the soulful melodies that echo through the lounge, transforming your nightcap into a harmonious blend of libations and live music, creating an atmosphere where every note is a tribute to Manhattan's musical legacy.

> **Crafted Cocktails with a Twist**: The nightcap menu at The Roxy Hotel features crafted cocktails with a twist. Mixologists here infuse creativity into every concoction, ensuring that your nightcap is a memorable experience, where traditional classics meet inventive innovation.

> **TriBeCa's Nighttime Enchantment**: TriBeCa's nighttime enchantment adds an extra layer of allure to your nightcap experience. The neighborhood's intimate streets and hidden gems create an atmosphere where each sip is a journey into the heart of Manhattan's nocturnal mystique.

> **The Legacy of Lower Manhattan**: As you enjoy your nightcap at The Roxy, you're embracing the legacy of Lower Manhattan. The historic streets and modern skyline serve as a testament to the city's resilience and spirit, reminding you that every nightcap is a celebration of Manhattan's enduring legacy.

As we venture further into "A Nightcap at The Roxy Hotel," we intertwine our exploration with the city's iconic landmarks, where each nightcap becomes a toast to Manhattan's nocturnal majesty. These libations are not just drinks; they are expressions of Manhattan's vibrant nightlife, where tradition meets innovation under the starry canopy.

EAT LIKE AN A-LISTER

Completed Tasks: Nightcap Activities

Action Items: Intentions and Thoughts

Action Items: Intentions and Thoughts

Manhattan's Midnight Indulgences: Guilt-Free Treats for After Hours

Manhattan—a city where the magic truly begins when the clock strikes twelve. In this metropolis of endless wonder, night isn't just the end of the day; it's the beginning of a tantalizing tale filled with temptations, treasures, and tastes. And in this nocturnal playground, it isn't just about satisfying hunger; it's about indulging—with grace, glamour, and an irresistible sense of glee.

Now envision: You're meandering along the moonlit lanes of the West Village, drawing glances, not from the shimmer of your shoes, but the seductive scent of the treat you hold. That, dearest, is the Manhattan Midnight Mystique, a culinary secret that is as savory as it is sweet, crafted with care, character, and a whisper of midnight charm.

In this delightful chapter of The Manhattan Diaries, we'll dive deep into the after-dark delights of the Big Apple. From velvety vegan chocolates that melt in the mouth to airy macarons that promise a dance of flavors, you'll unravel the art of midnight munching that's as light on the conscience as it is on the palate.

But it's not just about the bites. It's about the ambiance, the allure, the atmosphere. It's about slipping into the rhythm of Manhattan's moonlit melodies, feeding not just the body but the soul. It's about savoring both the sparkle of the city's glitzy cafes and the solace of its hidden dessert dens, capturing the essence of Manhattan's nocturnal nuances.

Come with me, as we saunter through the city's silent streets, sampling the sumptuous snacks that serenade the senses. Because, darling, in Manhattan, every bite after dark isn't just food—it's an enchanting epilogue to your day's story. Prepare to be entranced, for the city beckons with its bewitching bites. Welcome to The Manhattan Diaries—where your midnight morsel can be as mesmerizing as the city's moonlit moods.

127

Secrets of the Midnight Chocolate Alchemy

In the enchanting depths of Manhattan's midnight hours, a world of chocolate alchemy awaits those who seek indulgence beyond the ordinary. "Secrets of the Midnight Chocolate Alchemy" invites you to a culinary journey where artisanal chocolates, crafted with precision and passion, tantalize the senses and ignite the imagination. Picture this, darlings: silky, guilt-free chocolates melting on your tongue, created by master chocolatiers who infuse each bite with Manhattan's sophistication and allure. From velvety caramels to couture-inspired truffles, every piece of midnight chocolate is more than a treat; it's a celebration of art, luxury, and the spirit of the city that never sleeps. Join us as we uncover these sweet secrets, where cocoa meets creativity against the dazzling backdrop of Manhattan's iconic skyline.

➢ **Velvet Temptations**: Crafting Guilt-Free Midnight Chocolates: Delve into the world of artisanal midnight chocolates that are as sinfully delicious as they are ethically indulgent. Discover the secrets behind crafting these velvety temptations that melt in the mouth, tantalizing your taste buds without burdening your conscience.

➢ **The Midnight Chocolate Studio: Where Dreams Are Coated in Cocoa**: Journey into the heart of Manhattan's chocolatier studios, where talented artisans transform cocoa into midnight masterpieces. Explore the ambiance of these decadent workshops and experience how each truffle and bonbon is a work of art worthy of the city's creative spirit.

➢ **A Night of Chocolate and City Lights**: As you savor these midnight chocolates, let's savor the beauty of Manhattan's skyline. From the twinkling lights of Times Square to the iconic Empire State Building, the city's landmarks provide the perfect backdrop for a night of chocolate indulgence.

> **Manhattan's Chocolate Legacy**: Manhattan has a rich legacy when it comes to chocolate. Discover how this sweet treat has been woven into the city's history, from lavish society soirées to intimate chocolate-themed gatherings that have left an indelible mark on Manhattan's culinary tapestry.

> **Honeyed Caramel Kisses**: The Art of Filling: Explore the delicate art of creating caramel-filled midnight chocolates that deliver a symphony of flavors with every bite. Uncover the meticulous techniques employed to infuse these sweet kisses with Manhattan's sophisticated essence.

> **Cocoa and Cocktails: Pairing Midnight Chocolates with Manhattan Mixology**: Dive into the world of chocolate and cocktail pairings, where the art of mixology meets the allure of midnight chocolates. Discover how expertly crafted drinks complement and enhance the flavors of these decadent treats.

> **Chocolate Haute Couture: Manhattan's Chocolatier Fashion**: Delight in the intersection of fashion and chocolate as Manhattan's renowned chocolatiers create chocolate designs that mirror the city's haute couture. From chocolate stilettos to edible evening gowns, these sweet creations elevate chocolate to the realm of high fashion.

> **Chocolate and Luck: Truffle Treasures in the Financial District**: Explore the Financial District's hidden gems, where you'll find truffle treasures that bring luck and delight to the city's power players. Indulge in these chocolate gems while absorbing the ambiance of Wall Street and its iconic Charging Bull.

As we continue our journey through the "Secrets of the Midnight Chocolate Alchemy," dear readers, let's savor the delightful artistry and flavors that Manhattan's chocolatiers offer, all while basking in the splendor of the city's landmarks.

Completed Tasks: Midnight Chocolate Activities

Inspirational Quote

THE MEANING I PICKED, THE ONE THAT CHANGED MY LIFE: OVERCOME
FEAR, BEHOLD WONDER. — Richard Bach

Action Items: Intentions and Thoughts

Midnight Macarons: A Symphony of Flavors Under the Stars

In Manhattan's dazzling nightlife, "Midnight Macarons: A Symphony of Flavors Under the Stars" invites you to indulge in macarons that are as luxurious as they are delicious. Imagine savoring lavender, pistachio, and salted caramel treats on chic rooftops with views of iconic landmarks like the Chrysler Building. Each macaron becomes an edible masterpiece, capturing the city's essence in every bite. Join us as we explore this magical world where flavor and artistry meet under Manhattan's twinkling sky.

➢ **Macaron Magic**: Crafting Midnight's Edible Jewels: Enter the enchanting world of macaron-making, where delicate almond meringue cookies are transformed into edible jewels. Uncover the secrets of crafting these petite Parisian treats that offer a symphony of flavors beneath the Manhattan night sky.

➢ **The Flavor Palette: A Midnight Sonata of Tastes**: Explore the diverse flavors that dance within these midnight macarons. From classic French fillings like lavender and pistachio to contemporary Manhattan-inspired creations like matcha and salted caramel, every bite is a harmonious blend of taste and luxury.

➢ **Rooftop Revelry: Savoring Macarons with a View**: Indulge in macaron soirées at Manhattan's chic rooftop venues, where the glittering city skyline provides the backdrop for your sweet symphony. Experience the fusion of flavors and the panoramic views of iconic landmarks like the Chrysler Building.

➢ **Macaron Masterpieces: Artistry Meets Dessert**: Delve into the artistry behind crafting macaron masterpieces that pay homage to Manhattan's iconic landmarks. From macaron interpretations of the Statue of Liberty to the Brooklyn Bridge, these edible creations capture the essence of the city's architectural wonders.

➤ **Macaron Magic: Crafting Midnight's Edible Jewels**: Enter the enchanting world of macaron-making, where delicate almond meringue cookies are transformed into edible jewels. Uncover the secrets of crafting these petite Parisian treats that offer a symphony of flavors beneath the Manhattan night sky.

➤ **The Flavor Palette: A Midnight Sonata of Tastes**: Explore the diverse flavors that dance within these midnight macarons. From classic French fillings like lavender and pistachio to contemporary Manhattan-inspired creations like matcha and salted caramel, every bite is a harmonious blend of taste and luxury.

➤ **Rooftop Revelry: Savoring Macarons with a View**: Indulge in macaron soirées at Manhattan's chic rooftop venues, where the glittering city skyline provides the backdrop for your sweet symphony. Experience the fusion of flavors and the panoramic views of iconic landmarks like the Chrysler Building.

➤ **Macaron Masterpieces: Artistry Meets Dessert**: Delve into the artistry behind crafting macaron masterpieces that pay homage to Manhattan's iconic landmarks. From macaron interpretations of the Statue of Liberty to the Brooklyn Bridge, these edible creations capture the essence of the city's architectural wonders.

As we savor the "Midnight Macarons: A Symphony of Flavors Under the Stars," dear readers, let's remember that every macaron is not just a dessert but a luxurious work of art. In the world of Manhattan's culinary delights, where macarons become a symphony of flavors, we find ourselves immersed in both the artistry of the pastry chefs and the breathtaking beauty of the city's landmarks.

Completed Tasks: Midnight Macarons Activities

Inspirational Quote

OUR IDEALS ARE OUR BETTER SELVES. — Amos Bronson Alcott

Action Items: Intentions and Thoughts

The Allure of Moonlit Dessert Dens

In the heart of Manhattan's midnight magic, a world of hidden dessert dens awaits those who crave a taste of indulgence after dark. "The Allure of Moonlit Dessert Dens" invites you to explore these enchanting spots, where decadent sweets are enjoyed under the soft glow of the city's moonlit skyline. These late-night sanctuaries blend culinary artistry with sophisticated ambiance, offering treats like edible-gold sundaes, chocolate-champagne pairings, and pastries that feel like a work of art. Each dessert den, from cozy West Village nooks to elegant rooftop hideaways, transforms dessert into a luxurious escape, capturing the essence of Manhattan's charm. Join us as we uncover the magic of these midnight indulgences, where every bite is a moment of pure Manhattan allure.

> ➢ **Late-Night Luxuries: Moonlit Dessert Escapes**: Step into the world of Manhattan's hidden dessert dens, where the allure of late-night indulgence beckons. These enchanting eateries, illuminated by the soft glow of moonlight, offer a haven for those seeking sweet solace amidst the city's hustle and bustle.

> ➢ **Midnight Menu Magic: Decadence Under the Stars**: Delight in the enchanting midnight menus that these dessert dens curate. From exquisite sundaes adorned with edible gold to innovative pastries that redefine dessert, every bite is a journey into the realms of indulgence and sophistication.

> ➢ **Urban Oasis: Dessert Dens Amidst Manhattan's Majesty**: Explore dessert dens nestled within the heart of Manhattan's iconic neighborhoods. Whether it's a charming West Village cafe or a hidden gem in the Upper East Side, each location offers an intimate escape where desserts become an art form.

> ➢ **Champagne and Chocolate Dreams: Pairing Luxury with Dessert**: Indulge in the decadent pairing of champagne and

chocolate, a match made in dessert heaven. These dessert dens offer a curated selection of bubbly beverages that elevate the dessert experience to new heights.

➢ **Midnight Muse: Dessert as Creative Inspiration**: Discover how these moonlit dessert dens have become a muse for artists, writers, and creatives. Explore the intimate corners where the city's artistic soul finds solace and inspiration amidst delectable confections.

➢ **Artistic Ambiance: Dessert Dens as Gallery Spaces**: Immerse yourself in the artistic ambiance of these dessert dens, where the decor and presentation of desserts are akin to works of art. Explore how the aesthetic allure of these establishments complements the culinary delights.

➢ **Midnight Conversations: Dessert and the Language of Love:** Uncover the romantic allure of late-night dessert conversations, where couples and friends gather to share sweet moments under the starry Manhattan sky. These dessert dens serve as intimate settings for heartfelt connections and cherished memories.

➢ **Manhattan Moonlight Magic: Dessert Den Locations Revealed**: Get insider insights into the enchanting locations of these dessert dens, carefully chosen to immerse diners in the magic of Manhattan's moonlit nights. From hidden courtyards to rooftop terraces, each venue is a testament to the city's unique charm.

As we continue to explore "The Allure of Moonlit Dessert Dens," dear readers, let's savor the creative inspiration, artistic ambiance, romantic encounters, and the captivating locations that make these hidden gems a quintessential part of Manhattan's culinary landscape.

Completed Tasks: Moonlit Desserts Activities

Inspirational Quote

NO MATTER WHAT PEOPLE TELL YOU; WORDS AND IDEAS CAN CHANGE THE WORLD. — Robin Williams

Action Items: Intentions and Thoughts

EAT LIKE AN A-LISTER

Midnight Munching with a Side of Style

In the city that truly never sleeps, "Midnight Munching with a Side of Style" takes us into Manhattan's glamorous world of late-night dining, where culinary excellence meets high fashion. Picture this: chic venues illuminated by city lights, fashionable midnight bites paired with live jazz, and an atmosphere brimming with cosmopolitan flair. Here, style is as essential as the menu, and each venue, from rooftop terraces to intimate lounges, offers a uniquely curated night out. Join us as we explore the elegance of Manhattan after dark, where midnight feasts are a blend of flavor, fashion, and the city's iconic charm.

➢ **Manhattan After Dark: Where Style Meets the Midnight Hour**: Dive into the glamorous world of Manhattan's midnight munching scene, where style isn't just a choice; it's a way of life. These late-night hotspots offer a delectable combination of culinary excellence and cosmopolitan flair.

➢ **Midnight Elegance: Savoring the Night with Flair**: Indulge in the art of midnight elegance as you savor exquisite bites and beverages. Discover how these fashionable venues elevate late-night dining to a chic social experience, where every moment is an opportunity to dazzle.

➢ **Fashion-Forward Feasts: Late-Night Haunts of the Well-Heeled**: Explore the late-night haunts frequented by Manhattan's well-heeled denizens. From celebrity sightings to runway-inspired decor, these establishments effortlessly blend haute cuisine with high fashion.

➢ **Midnight Stars and City Lights: Manhattan's Iconic Backdrop**: Immerse yourself in the enchanting ambiance created by Manhattan's iconic landmarks. Whether you're dining under the starry canopy of Central Park or enjoying city views from a rooftop terrace, these settings add an extra layer of allure to your midnight munching experience.

➢ **Late-Night Fashionistas**: Manhattan's Midnight Wardrobe: Explore how Manhattan's fashionistas curate their late-night wardrobes, effortlessly blending comfort and style for their midnight escapades. Discover the fashion trends that define the city's after-hours glamour.

➢ **Musical Notes and Midnight Melodies**: Delve into the musical choices that set the mood for late-night dining. From live jazz performances to curated playlists, these venues ensure that every note complements the culinary symphony, making your midnight feast an auditory delight.

➢ **Midnight Soirees: Chic Events Beyond Dinner**: Uncover the allure of midnight soirees and exclusive events hosted by these fashionable late-night hotspots. Whether it's a themed masquerade ball or an intimate wine tasting, these gatherings add an extra layer of sophistication to your midnight adventures.

➢ **Nighttime City Escapes: Manhattan's Midnight Transit**: Navigate the city's midnight terrain as we discuss the various transportation options available for those seeking stylish late-night dining. From chauffeur-driven cars to iconic yellow taxis, getting to your midnight destination is as much a part of the experience as the dining itself.

As we venture into "Midnight Munching with a Side of Style," dear readers, let's embrace the cosmopolitan charm, midnight elegance, fashion-forward feasts, and the iconic Manhattan backdrop that make late-night dining a glamorous affair in the city that never sleeps.

Completed Tasks: Midnight Munching Style Activities

Inspirational Quote

TOO MANY COMPANIES WANT THEIR BRANDS TO REFLECT SOME IDEALIZED, PERFECTED IMAGE OF THEMSELVES. AS A CONSEQUENCE, THEIR BRANDS ACQUIRE NO TEXTURE, NO CHARACTER, AND NO PUBLIC TRUST. — Richard Branson

MANHATTAN'S MIDNIGHT INDULGENCES

Action Items: Intentions and Thoughts

Action Items: Intentions and Thoughts

West Village Wellness:
Superfoods to Keep You Glowing from Within

8

Manhattan, a city pulsating with electrifying energy, is constantly in search of the next big thing. Yet, amidst its whirlwind chaos and charm, the historic West Village stands as an enclave of tranquility, with health-conscious havens that beckon the discerning and the dedicated. In this neighborhood of cobbled corners, it isn't just about nourishing the body; it's about feeding the soul—with elegance, élan, and a splash of ethereal energy.

Visualize: You're strolling down Bleecker Street, a radiant aura enveloping you. Onlookers don't merely admire the silkiness of your scarf, but the luminosity of your skin, the spark in your eyes. That, my dear, is the West Village Wellness Waltz, a rhythm that speaks of purity, vitality, and an undying zest for life.

In this refreshing chapter of The Manhattan Diaries, we're going to explore the culinary treasures that offer more than just a feast for the eyes. From emerald green matcha lattes that promise an antioxidant punch, to chia seed puddings that glisten with promises of omega-3 goodness, you'll learn to nourish your body in a way that shines through every pore, every glance, every smile.

But, as always, it's more than just the meal. It's the magic that Manhattan weaves into its very fabric. It's about being in sync with the rhythm of the West Village, where history mingles with hipster vibes. Embracing the cafes that offer solace from the skyscrapers, and sinking into the embrace of wellness that envelops this little nook of New York.

So, accompany me on a journey where every bite is a promise of rejuvenation, every sip a symphony of nutrients. Because, darling, in the West Village, your glow isn't just about the right highlighter—it's about the radiance that comes from within. Prepare for a transformative trek, for the city has secrets that can elevate you, body and soul. Welcome to The

Manhattan Diaries—where your inner vitality can rival the sparkle of Times Square.

Glowing from Within: The Art of West Village Wellness

Amidst the bustling cityscape of Manhattan, the West Village emerges as a tranquil sanctuary where well-being becomes an art form, and inner radiance is nurtured with grace and style. Imagine strolling along the historic streets of Bleecker and Grove, a radiant aura enveloping you, catching the admiring glances of passersby who are drawn not only to your chic attire but also to the luminosity of your skin and the twinkle in your eyes. This, my dear readers, is the West Village Wellness Waltz, where purity, vitality, and an unbridled zest for life take center stage. In this captivating chapter of The Manhattan Diaries, we'll embark on a journey to explore the culinary treasures and wellness havens that define the West Village experience.

➢ **Nourishment Elixirs**: Sip your way to vitality with nutrient-packed smoothie bowls and herbal teas that soothe the senses. In West Village, it's not just a beverage; it's a revitalizing ritual that invigorates your spirit for the day ahead.

➢ **Farm-to-Table Charm**: Discover how the West Village's unwavering commitment to locally sourced produce and artisanal ingredients shapes its farm-to-table dining experiences. Here, every bite is a celebration of freshness and flavor, and it's an embodiment of the neighborhood's culinary ethos.

➢ **Wellness Retreats**: Explore the serene wellness havens tucked away within the neighborhood, offering respite from the city's relentless pace. In these sanctuaries, you can rejuvenate your body and soul, embracing the West Village's dedication to holistic well-being.

➢ **Morning Rituals**: Delve into the morning practices embraced by West Village locals, setting the tone for a day filled with well-being.

It's a sacred time when the neighborhood's charm truly shines, and you'll find yourself effortlessly aligning with the peaceful rhythms of this enclave.

➤ **Hidden Green Oases**: Uncover the secret gardens and serene parks hidden within the West Village, offering peaceful spots for meditation, yoga, or simply basking in the tranquility of nature, all while staying close to the heart of the city.

➤ **Spa Escapes**: Indulge in the neighborhood's exclusive spa experiences that blend luxury and holistic wellness. From rejuvenating facials to soothing massages, these wellness retreats offer an escape from the urban hustle and a chance to pamper yourself in style.

➤ **Artisanal Wellness Markets**: Dive into the neighborhood's vibrant wellness markets, where local artisans showcase their handcrafted wellness products, from organic skincare to herbal remedies. It's a sensory journey through the West Village's commitment to holistic living.

➤ **Evening Serenity**: Experience the West Village's transformation as night falls, where the streets are illuminated with a soft glow, and cozy candlelit cafes invite you to unwind. It's an enchanting way to conclude your day in this haven of well-being.

In the heart of Manhattan, the West Village's dedication to inner vitality, serene sanctuaries, and a harmonious way of life makes it a neighborhood like no other. As we explore these aspects in the West Village, remember that here, your glow isn't just skin deep; it's a reflection of the neighborhood's unwavering commitment to well-being. Prepare to be enchanted by the West Village's radiant charm and its transformative effects on both body and soul. Welcome to The Manhattan Diaries, where your inner vitality shines as brightly as the city lights.

Completed Tasks: Wellness Waltz Activities

(lined writing space)

Inspirational Quote

THE BOOKS THAT HELP YOU MOST ARE THOSE WHICH MAKE YOU THINK THE MOST. THE HARDEST WAY OF LEARNING IS THAT OF EASY READING; BUT A GREAT BOOK THAT COMES FROM A GREAT THINKER IS A SHIP OF THOUGHT, DEEP FREIGHTED WITH TRUTH AND BEAUTY. — Pablo Neruda

Action Items: Intentions and Thoughts

Nourishment Elixirs: Sipping Your Way to Vitality

Nestled within Manhattan's vibrant heart, the historic West Village offers a serene haven amid the city's ceaseless pace. In this chapter of The Manhattan Diaries, we delve into the neighborhood's devotion to holistic living. From invigorating matcha lattes to nourishing smoothies and delightful chia seed puddings, we explore elixirs that promise rejuvenation and vitality. Join me on a journey through the West Village's dedication to well-being, where each sip is a step toward inner radiance. Welcome to a world where your vitality shines as bright as the city lights, an oasis in Manhattan's bustling landscape.

➢ **Matcha Magic**: Dive into the world of vibrant green matcha lattes, where tradition meets trendiness. These antioxidant-rich elixirs promise an invigorating sip that kickstarts your day, a perfect complement to the city's energetic pulse.

➢ **Fresh-Pressed Juices**: Explore the West Village's array of juice bars offering freshly squeezed elixirs bursting with vitamins and nutrients. These colorful concoctions promise to detoxify and energize, making them a favorite choice for health-conscious Manhattanites.

➢ **Avocado Enchantments**: Discover the West Village's love affair with avocados in the form of creamy, nutrient-packed smoothies. These luscious blends are not only delicious but also brimming with healthy fats and essential nutrients, elevating your well-being with each sip.

➢ **Chia Seed Wonders**: Delight in chia seed puddings that glisten with promises of omega-3 goodness. These delightful creations are both nourishing and indulgent, embodying the West Village's commitment to holistic living.

➤ **Golden Turmeric Lattes**: Embrace the warmth of golden turmeric lattes, a favorite among West Village wellness enthusiasts. Rich with anti-inflammatory benefits, these vibrant drinks soothe and rejuvenate, making them the perfect comfort elixir for busy Manhattan days.

➤ **Herbal Infusions and Adaptogen Teas**: Discover the range of herbal infusions and adaptogen teas that cater to stress relief and balance. These potent brews, crafted from nature's finest herbs, bring calming vibes and an earthy depth to your well-being journey.

➤ **Coconut Kefir and Probiotic Sips**: Sip on coconut kefir and probiotic drinks that nourish your gut health. These creamy, tangy elixirs are packed with live cultures, supporting digestion and strengthening the immune system with each sip.

➤ **Berry Bliss Smoothies**: Dive into berry-packed smoothies rich in antioxidants and vitamins. These vibrant, fruity elixirs blend strawberries, blueberries, and goji berries to create a delicious, energizing burst of color and nutrition.

➤ **Collagen-Boosted Blends**: Indulge in collagen-infused beverages designed to support skin, hair, and nail health. These beauty-boosting elixirs are a West Village favorite for their nourishing properties that bring a glow from the inside out.

As we navigate the West Village's world of nourishment elixirs, we'll realize that here, vitality isn't just a goal; it's a way of life. Each sip and swallow is a step towards inner radiance, and each wellness cafe visit is an opportunity to embrace a harmonious existence. So, let's raise our glasses to the West Village's dedication to well-being, where the elixirs are as transformative as the city's iconic skyline. Welcome to The Manhattan Diaries, where your journey to vitality is as vibrant as a New York sunrise.

Completed Tasks: Nourishment Elixirs Activities

Inspirational Quote

SPACE IS AN INSPIRATIONAL CONCEPT THAT ALLOWS YOU TO DREAM BIG.
— Peter Diamandis

Action Items: Intentions and Thoughts

EAT LIKE AN A-LISTER

Farm-to-Table Charm: Culinary Delights from Local Producers

Amidst the hustle and bustle of Manhattan's urban landscape, the West Village stands as a sanctuary of farm-to-table dining, where the culinary scene thrives on the elegance of locally sourced, seasonal ingredients. In this tantalizing chapter of The Manhattan Diaries, we embark on a culinary journey through the West Village's dedication to freshness and flavor. From charming cheese shops that transport you to pastoral landscapes to cozy bistros serving dishes crafted from the region's finest, we'll unravel the farm-to-table charm that defines this neighborhood's dining culture. So, let's explore the West Village's culinary delights, where each bite is a tribute to the synergy of nature and city living. Welcome to a world where local producers take center stage amidst the iconic Manhattan skyline.

- ➢ **Artisanal Eateries**: The West Village is home to an array of intimate eateries and restaurants that celebrate the bond between chefs and local farmers. Seasonal menus are crafted with precision, offering dishes that mirror the ever-changing bounty of the region.

- ➢ **Neighborhood Farmers' Markets**: Explore the vibrant farmers' markets that dot the neighborhood's charming streets. These bustling marketplaces offer an array of farm-fresh produce, artisanal cheeses, and handcrafted goods, providing a sensory experience like no other.

- ➢ **Sustainable Seafood Selections**: Delight your palate with sustainable seafood options at renowned seafood restaurants in the West Village. Here, a commitment to ocean-friendly sourcing is paired with culinary artistry to bring you dishes that are both delectable and ecologically responsible.

- ➢ **Seasonal Sips**: Elevate your libation experience by visiting the neighborhood's bars and cocktail lounges, where mixologists showcase local spirits and seasonal ingredients in their concoctions.

Each sip is a toast to the West Village's farm-to-table philosophy, served with a dash of creativity and flair.

➤ **Market Fresh Delights**: Immerse yourself in the West Village's vibrant farmers' markets, where local artisans and growers gather to showcase their freshest, seasonal treasures. Stroll through the stalls brimming with colorful produce, handcrafted cheeses, and artisanal goods, all sourced from nearby farms. Let the market's lively atmosphere envelop you as you select the finest ingredients for your farm-to-table feast.

➤ **Sustainable Seafood Feasts**: Dive into the neighborhood's sustainable seafood scene, where you can savor exquisite dishes crafted from the bounty of nearby waters. Explore local seafood restaurants that take pride in offering ocean-friendly options, ensuring that every bite not only delights your palate but also supports responsible fishing practices and marine conservation.

➤ **Craft Beverage Adventures**: Immerse yourself in the West Village's craft beverage scene, from neighborhood breweries and cideries to cozy wine bars featuring regional vintages.

➤ **Local Food Festivals**: Don't miss the neighborhood's food festivals, celebrating seasonal flavors and culinary traditions while fostering a sense of community and local pride.

In the heart of Manhattan's West Village, farm-to-table dining takes center stage, where locally sourced, seasonal ingredients shine. This chapter of The Manhattan Diaries invites you to savor the enchanting world of the West Village, where farms and producers shape culinary creations. Whether dining in eateries, exploring farmers' markets, indulging in sustainable seafood, or sipping seasonal beverages, each meal reflects the vibrant tapestry of this iconic New York neighborhood. Welcome to the West Village, where farm-to-table dining is a testament to Manhattan's enduring culinary allure.

Completed Tasks: Farm to Table Activities

Inspirational Quote

BRAND IS NOT A PRODUCT, THAT'S FOR SURE; IT'S NOT ONE ITEM. IT'S AN IDEA, IT'S A THEORY, IT'S A MEANING, IT'S HOW YOU CARRY YOURSELF. IT'S ASPIRATIONAL, IT'S INSPIRATIONAL. — Kevin Plank

Action Items: Intentions and Thoughts

EAT LIKE AN A-LISTER

Wellness Retreats in the Heart of Manhattan

Amidst the bustling streets and towering skyscrapers of Manhattan, a hidden world of wellness and tranquility awaits those seeking a respite from the urban hustle. In the heart of this concrete jungle, wellness retreats offer an oasis of serenity, providing a sanctuary where you can rejuvenate your mind, body, and spirit. Picture yourself amidst the city's energetic rhythms, yet enveloped in a cocoon of calm. That, my dear, is the Wellness Wonderland of Manhattan—a place where self-care takes center stage, and where the pursuit of inner harmony meets the vibrant pulse of the city.

- ➤ **Urban Sanctuaries**: Discover urban sanctuaries tucked away in the midst of Manhattan's lively neighborhoods. These havens of tranquility offer yoga studios, meditation spaces, and wellness centers where you can escape the city's frenetic pace and embark on a journey of self-discovery and renewal.

- ➤ **Mindful Movement**: Immerse yourself in the world of mindful movement, where the city's vibrant energy fuses with holistic practices. From rooftop yoga sessions with breathtaking skyline views to outdoor tai chi classes in serene parks, you'll find opportunities to align your body, mind, and spirit amidst the city's dynamic landscape.

- ➤ **Spa Escapes**: Treat yourself to luxurious spa experiences that rival those of any global destination. Manhattan's top spas offer an array of rejuvenating treatments, from traditional massages to innovative therapies, all designed to pamper your senses and restore your inner balance.

- ➤ **Nutrient-Rich Dining**: Nourish your body with nutrient-rich cuisine at wellness-focused restaurants and cafes. Explore menus that feature locally sourced, organic ingredients, and innovative dishes that not only tantalize your taste buds but also support your overall well-being.

➤ **Holistic Retreats**: Embark on holistic retreats within the city, where you can immerse yourself in transformative workshops, wellness seminars, and immersive experiences. These retreats provide an opportunity to deepen your connection with yourself and like-minded individuals, fostering a sense of community and self-discovery amidst Manhattan's vibrant backdrop.

➤ **Outdoor Wellness Adventures**: Experience the beauty of Manhattan's natural landscapes through outdoor wellness adventures. Join guided hikes in nearby parks, practice yoga on the waterfront, or partake in forest bathing sessions to connect with nature while revitalizing your body and mind.

➤ **Mindfulness Workshops**: Engage in mindfulness workshops and meditation sessions that teach you how to incorporate mindfulness practices into your daily life. These workshops provide valuable tools for managing stress, enhancing focus, and promoting overall well-being, all within the heart of the city that never sleeps.

As you delve into the world of wellness retreats in Manhattan, you'll find that this city's allure extends far beyond its iconic landmarks and bustling streets. Here, in these serene enclaves, you can truly connect with the essence of the city, finding inner peace and balance while embracing the energy that makes Manhattan the extraordinary place that it is. So, dear reader, prepare to embark on a journey of self-discovery and rejuvenation in the heart of Manhattan, where every breath is a step toward wellness, and every moment is an opportunity to embrace the vibrant spirit of the city. Welcome to The Manhattan Diaries—where your path to inner harmony is as enchanting as the city itself.

Completed Tasks: Wellness Retreats Activities

Inspirational Quote

LEE'S GREAT GIFTS ARE TEACHING AND INSPIRATIONAL GUIDANCE, NOT ADMINISTRATION AND MANAGEMENT. — Cheryl Crawford

Action Items: Intentions and Thoughts

Morning Rituals and Wellness: Starting Your Day Right

In the city that never sleeps, mornings in Manhattan are a symphony of opportunity and energy. From sunrise yoga sessions along the Hudson River to serene meditation on rooftop terraces with iconic skyline views, the heart of Manhattan pulses with wellness possibilities at the break of dawn. Join us on a journey through Manhattan's morning rituals, where well-being meets the city's vibrant spirit. Whether you're a local seeking serenity amidst the urban hustle or a visitor eager to embrace the city's wellness offerings, these morning practices will set the tone for an inspiring day in the Big Apple.

➢ **Sunrise Yoga on the Hudson**: Begin your day with a picturesque sunrise yoga session on the banks of the Hudson River. With the Statue of Liberty as your backdrop and the gentle lapping of the river's waves as your soundtrack, it's a serene way to invigorate both body and soul.

➢ **Rooftop Meditation at Dawn**: Some of Manhattan's chicest hotels offer rooftop meditation experiences at sunrise. As you gaze out over the city's iconic skyline, you'll find a sense of tranquility amidst the urban hustle and bustle.

➢ **Healthy Breakfast at a Stylish Café**: Fuel your body with a healthy breakfast at one of Manhattan's trendy wellness cafes. From acai bowls bursting with antioxidants to avocado toast paired with artisanal coffee, these cafes offer a delicious start to your day.

➢ **Soul-Nourishing Walk in Central Park**: Explore the lush serenity of Central Park with a morning walk or jog. The park's winding pathways, serene lakes, and lush greenery provide an oasis of calm amidst the city's vibrant energy.

➢ **Mindfulness and Gratitude Journaling**: Embrace mindfulness and gratitude by journaling your thoughts and intentions for the day.

With the city's iconic skyline as your backdrop, it's a moment to reflect on your aspirations and embrace the opportunities Manhattan has to offer.

➢ **Morning Juice Cleanse**: Manhattan's juice bars offer a variety of rejuvenating morning elixirs. From cold-pressed green juices to ginger shots, these elixirs provide a refreshing boost to start the day.

➢ **Wellness Workshops and Seminars**: Attend wellness workshops and seminars led by experts in the field. These sessions cover topics such as stress management, mindfulness practices, and holistic nutrition, helping you prioritize your well-being amidst the city's fast pace.

➢ **SoulCycle and Spin Classes**: Join a high-energy SoulCycle or spin class at one of Manhattan's premier fitness studios. The camaraderie and motivation of a group workout, set against the city's iconic skyline, can be invigorating.

➢ **Spa and Self-Care Rituals**: Treat yourself to a spa or self-care ritual that pampers your body and mind. Manhattan's luxury spas offer a range of treatments, from rejuvenating facials to therapeutic massages, ensuring you start your day feeling refreshed and renewed.

➢ **Inspirational Sunrise Views**: Catching the sunrise from iconic Manhattan locations like the Brooklyn Bridge or the High Line Park can be an inspiring way to start your day.

In Manhattan, mornings are a canvas of wellness and vitality, offering a blend of opportunities to kickstart your day. From yoga sessions by the Hudson to rooftop meditation with iconic views, the city's sunrise rituals harmonize wellbeing with its vibrant spirit. Whether you're a local seeking serenity or a visitor embracing wellness, these practices will inspire your day in the Big Apple.

Completed Tasks: Morning Wellness Ritual Activities

Inspirational Quote

I LOOK UP TO A STRONG WOMAN; MAYBE THAT'S WHY I FELL FOR GAGA. SHE WORKS INCREDIBLY HARD AND IS VERY STRONG AND INSPIRATIONAL LIKE MOM, WITH A GREAT WORK ETHIC. — Taylor Kinney

Action Items: Intentions and Thoughts

Action Items: Intentions and Thoughts

9

East Side Elixirs: Smoothies and Juices the Celebs Won't Stop Talking About

Manhattan, a city shimmering under a canopy of bright lights and even brighter stars. But while the skyline dazzles, there's another shimmer that's drawing everyone's attention: the radiant health emanating from the crème de la crème of the Upper East Side. Yes, in a borough renowned for its posh penthouses and swanky soirees, the latest talk isn't just about the latest couture but about a refreshing concoction in a glass. In Manhattan, where the race never stops, it's about fueling your journey—with flair, finesse, and a splash of fruity freshness.

Visualize: You're sauntering past Park Avenue, and the murmur isn't about the Chanel you're wearing but the vibrant green smoothie you're sipping. That, darling, is the East Side Elixir Elegance, a dance that speaks of health, opulence, and a commitment to only the finest.

In this invigorating chapter of The Manhattan Diaries, we delve deep into the world of verdant veggies and fabulous fruits, blended to perfection, served in style. From the A-list Avocado Ambrosia that promises a skin as smooth as silk to the Berry Blast Bonanza that's a paparazzi favorite, here you'll unveil the secret sips that the city's elite swear by.

However, remember, this isn't just about the taste or health benefits. It's the entire East Side experience. It's about sipping an elixir with the same elegance as you'd wear a Dior. Embracing both the glitz of the grand ballrooms and the greens of these goblets, mastering the balance between indulgence and wellness.

So, come with me, as we discover the secret spots, the hidden haunts, and the whispered recipes that are all the rage. Because, sweetheart, in the Upper East Side, sipping a smoothie isn't just about nutrition; it's about making a statement. Ready to immerse in the world of glamorous greens and ritzy reds? The city is pouring out its secrets, and every drop is worth its weight in gold. Welcome to The Manhattan Diaries—where your drink is as enigmatic as the tales of the city.

Upper East Side Elixirs: A Taste of Manhattan's High Life

In the Upper East Side of Manhattan, where every block tells a story of opulence and elegance, a new trend is taking the elite by storm: East Side Elixirs. These are not just drinks; they're statements of taste, health, and sophistication. Picture this: You're strolling along Madison Avenue, and it's not your designer handbag that turns heads but the vibrant elixir in your hand. This, darling, is the East Side Elixir Elegance—an ode to wellness, luxury, and a commitment to the finest things in life.

➢ **A-List Avocado Ambrosia**: Discover the smoothie that promises a complexion as flawless as a couture gown. Explore the hidden gems of the Upper East Side where you'll find these secret spots, hidden haunts, and whispered recipes.

➢ **Berry Blast Bonanza**: Unveil the paparazzies favorite juice that's taking the Upper East Side by storm. Peek into the exclusive locales of Manhattan where you can uncover these secret spots, hidden haunts, and whispered recipes.

➢ **Glamorous Greens**: Explore the world of verdant veggies and fabulous fruits, blended to perfection. Delve into the discreet establishments throughout the city, where the secret spots, hidden haunts, and whispered recipes await.

➢ **Ritzy Reds**: Sip on the secret elixirs that the city's elite swear by for a dose of vitality and style. Uncover the mysterious venues in Manhattan where these secret spots, hidden haunts, and whispered recipes are guarded with care.

➢ **Society Sips**: Delve into the elite social circles of the Upper East Side, where exclusive events and gatherings are incomplete without

East Side Elixirs.   Uncover the upscale venues favored by Manhattan's high society, where the secret spots, hidden haunts, and whispered recipes are shared among the privileged few.

➢ **Health and Hedonism**: Explore the intriguing duality of the Upper East Side lifestyle, where residents balance their commitment to well-being with a taste for the exquisite. Venture into the wellness centers and luxury lounges where East Side Elixirs seamlessly merge health-consciousness and hedonism, revealing the secret spots, hidden haunts, and whispered recipes that epitomize this lifestyle.

➢ **Celebrity Sips**: Get a glimpse into the favored elixirs of Manhattan's A-list celebrities who call the Upper East Side their home. Visit the chic establishments where the stars indulge in East Side Elixirs, and uncover the secret spots, hidden haunts, and whispered recipes that cater to their discerning tastes.

➢ **Elixir Etiquette**: Learn the art of savoring East Side Elixirs with sophistication and grace. Discover the unspoken rules and rituals that accompany these drinks in Manhattan's high life, reflecting the culture of the Upper East Side and the secret spots, hidden haunts, and whispered recipes that define it.

However, it's not just about the taste or health benefits. It's about the entire East Side experience—a harmonious blend of elegance and indulgence. So, come with me as we uncover the secret spots, the hidden haunts, and the whispered recipes that are all the rage. Because, darling, in the Upper East Side, sipping a smoothie isn't just about nutrition; it's about making a statement. Ready to immerse in the world of glamorous greens and ritzy reds? The city is pouring out its secrets, and every drop is worth its weight in gold. Welcome to The Manhattan Diaries-where your drink is as enigmatic as the tales of the city.

Completed Tasks: Elixir Elegance Activities

Inspirational Quote

BETTER TO BE CALLED SOMETHING POSITIVE AND INSPIRATIONAL THAN SOMETHING NEGATIVE. — Donnie Yen

Action Items: Intentions and Thoughts

Sips of Celebrity Secrets: Iconic Smoothie Recipes from the Elite

In the glittering playground of Manhattan, where the pursuit of perfection is a way of life, there exists a hidden world of wellness secrets known only to the elite. Beyond the dazzling lights of Broadway and the opulence of Fifth Avenue, the city's upper echelons have mastered the art of sipping their way to vitality with iconic smoothie recipes. Picture yourself strolling down Madison Avenue, Where the conversation isn't about the latest fashion trends, but the glowing radiance achieved through a secret blend. Welcome to "Sips of Celebrity Secrets," a tantalizing chapter in The Manhattan Diaries, where we unlock the guarded recipes that keep the city's stars shining. From the private kitchens of A-list celebrities to the chicest health-conscious cafes, join us as we sip, savor, and spill the beans on the iconic smoothies that fuel the high life in Manhattan.

➤ **Celebrity Sips**: Step into the world of Manhattan's glitterati as we unveil the favorite smoothie recipes of A-list celebrities. Discover the secret ingredients and personal touches that keep them looking and feeling their best.

➤ **Chic Cafes and Hidden Gems**: Explore the upscale cafes and hidden gems of the city where these iconic smoothies are crafted to perfection. From charming neighborhood haunts to trendy wellness retreats, we'll take you to the places where the elite gather.

➤ **Behind Closed Doors**: Peek behind the curtains of private kitchens as we visit the homes of some of Manhattan's most renowned figures. Learn the exclusive recipes and rituals that have become part of their daily routines.

➤ **Sipping with Style:** Dive into the Upper East Side's sophisticated culture of health and wellness, where a smoothie isn't just a drink but a statement. From designer activewear to luxury fitness studios, discover the lifestyle that accompanies these iconic sips.

➤ **Culinary Collaborations**: Explore the unique collaborations between celebrity chefs and nutrition experts that have given rise to these iconic smoothie recipes. Delve into the innovative culinary techniques and cutting-edge ingredients that set them apart.

➤ **The Power of Superfoods**: Uncover the role of superfoods in Manhattan's smoothie culture. From acai to spirulina, learn how these nutrient-packed ingredients add a touch of prestige and health benefits to each blend.

➤ **Smoothie as Lifestyle**: Gain insights into how the elite incorporate these iconic smoothies into their daily routines. Discover the morning rituals and wellness practices that go hand in hand with sipping on these health-conscious concoctions.

➤ **The Manhattan Sip**: Elegance in Every Glass: Experience the art of presentation as we delve into the elegant aesthetics of these iconic smoothies. From exquisite glassware to artistic garnishes, witness how each sip becomes a work of culinary art in the city that never sleeps.

➤ **Midnight Detox: The Elite's Post-Event Ritual**: Discover the celebrity-approved detox smoothies that Manhattan's elite rely on after glitzy events and late-night soirées. These rejuvenating blends, featuring ingredients like activated charcoal, aloe vera, and ginger, are crafted to reset and refresh, restoring vitality for morning after.

In the heart of Manhattan, where every sip is a statement, join us in unraveling the secrets of these iconic smoothie recipes. From Madison Avenue to Central Park, we'll guide you through the city's landmarks while indulging in the flavors that define the elite's quest for health and vitality. Welcome to The Manhattan Diaries, where glamour, wellness, and sophistication converge in every delicious sip.

EAT LIKE AN A-LISTER

Completed Tasks: Iconic Smoothies Activities

Inspirational Quote

THE POWER OF POP CULTURE STORIES SHOULD NOT BE UNDERESTIMATED, AND THERE IS AN ENORMOUS POTENTIAL FOR INSPIRATIONAL STORIES THAT CAN HAVE A POSITIVE, TRANSFORMATIVE EFFECT ON OUR LIVES. — Anita Sarkeesian

Action Items: Intentions and Thoughts

Health Meets Glamour: The Upper East Side Wellness Lifestyle

In Manhattan's Upper East Side, where luxury meets wellness, a new lifestyle is blossoming, blending health with glamour and elegance. Here, living fabulously means radiating wellness as much as wearing designer attire. Welcome to the Upper East Side Wellness Whimsy, where vitality is the ultimate accessory. In this exclusive Manhattan Diaries chapter, we'll uncover the finest spa retreats, gourmet health dining, and secret wellness spots that embody this neighborhood's chic commitment to well-being.

➤ **Spa Sanctuaries**: Delve into the world of opulent wellness spas nestled among the Upper East Side's iconic landmarks. Discover how the elite unwind and rejuvenate with bespoke treatments and luxurious pampering.

➤ **Gourmet Wellness Dining**: Explore the haute cuisine of health-conscious dining in Manhattan's most prestigious restaurants. From farm-to-table delights to plant-based culinary extravaganzas, savor the flavors that define the Upper East Side's wellness scene.

➤ **Wellness Boutiques**: Step inside the upscale wellness boutiques that line Madison Avenue, offering everything from designer activewear to artisanal wellness products. Uncover the curated collections that cater to the neighborhood's health-savvy denizens.

➤ **Fitness Fusion**: Witness the fusion of fitness and fashion as we delve into the Upper East Side's innovative workout studios and wellness clubs. From rooftop yoga with a view to exclusive personal training, explore the ways the elite stay in shape.

➤ **Wellness Walks**: Wander through the historic streets and serene pockets of the Upper East Side, where every step becomes a mindful journey. Explore the neighborhood's hidden gardens and tranquil enclaves that offer respite from the city's hustle and bustle.

➤ **Holistic Retreats**: Uncover the wellness retreats and holistic centers that offer a haven of serenity amidst the urban chaos. Learn how the elite escape the city's frenetic pace to recharge their spirits and nourish their souls.

➤ **Wellness Wisdom**: Dive into the world of wellness experts and practitioners who call the Upper East Side home. Discover their secrets, from mindfulness techniques to holistic approaches, that keep the neighborhood's residents in top form.

➤ **Artistic Wellness**: Experience how the Upper East Side's artistic community incorporates wellness into their creative processes. Explore the galleries, studios, and performances that celebrate the harmonious blend of art and wellbeing in this cultural hub.

➤ **Beauty Elixirs: Sip Your Way to Radiance**: Discover the Upper East Side's favorite wellness cafes and juice bars, where beauty elixirs are crafted with superfoods, collagen, and adaptogens. These nutrient-rich beverages promise a radiant glow from the inside out, offering a delicious fusion of taste and vitality that complements the neighborhood's dedication to beauty and well-being.

➤ **Luxury Sleep Sanctuaries: Curated Rest for the Elite**: From sleep-optimizing bedding boutiques to exclusive relaxation therapies, these spaces redefine rest, catering to the neighborhood's discerning wellness seekers in pursuit of the perfect night's sleep.

Join us as we embark on a journey through this neighborhood where health meets glamour, and every step you take is a statement of self-care. In a landscape adorned with iconic landmarks and prestigious addresses, we'll reveal the secrets, stories, and sophistication that define the Upper East Side's wellness lifestyle. Welcome to The Manhattan Diaries, where well-being is the new luxury, and living vibrantly is the true art of existence.

EAT LIKE AN A-LISTER

Completed Tasks: Health and Glamour Activities

Inspirational Quote

I HAD HOPED WHEN MY LIFE WAS CHRONICLED, IT WOULD BE AN INSPIRATIONAL STORY. — Om Puri

Action Items: Intentions and Thoughts

The Art of Sipping: How to Enjoy Your Smoothie Like a Manhattanite

Amidst the relentless energy of Manhattan, the Upper East Side stands as an oasis of wellness and sophistication, where residents have elevated health to an art form. In this chapter of The Manhattan Diaries, we uncover the secrets of this wellness lifestyle, from exquisite smoothie recipes to morning rituals and serene settings, all against the backdrop of the city that never sleeps. Join us on a journey where each sip is a tribute to living well in Manhattan's most refined neighborhood.

➢ **The Elegance of Presentation**: Manhattan's elite know that sipping a smoothie is an art form. Discover how to garnish your glass with edible flowers, fresh fruit, or a sprinkle of superfoods, turning your daily ritual into a visual masterpiece.

➢ **Refined Ingredients**: Explore the Upper East Side's hidden gourmet grocers and specialty markets, where the elite source their premium ingredients. From organic berries to handcrafted almond milk, learn the secrets to creating a smoothie that's both delicious and nutritious.

➢ **Rituals of Rhythm**: Delve into the daily routines of Manhattan's wellness aficionados. Uncover the morning rituals and mindfulness practices that set the tone for a day of success and vitality, all while savoring your smoothie like a true insider.

➢ **Sips of Serenity**: From Central Park's lush landscapes to the chic cafes nestled along Museum Mile, sip your smoothie amidst iconic Manhattan landmarks. Discover how the Upper East Side's serene surroundings enhance the pleasure of every sip.

➢ **Smoothie Soirees**: Join the elite at exclusive smoothie gatherings in upscale Upper East Side apartments, where conversations flow as freely as the blended concoctions. Learn the etiquette of networking over nutrient-packed drinks, forging connections that power the city's success stories.

➤ **The Art of Morning Rituals**: Discover how Upper East Siders start their day with intention, incorporating meditation, yoga, and gratitude practices into their morning routines.

➤ **Serene Spots in the Concrete Jungle**: Explore the hidden parks and green spaces of the Upper East Side, offering residents a respite from the bustling city streets.

➤ **Nutrition for Radiance**: Delve into the gourmet, health-conscious dining options available in this neighborhood, where farm-to-table and sustainable cuisine take center stage.

➤ **Living Well in Luxury**: Uncover the exclusive wellness clubs and spas that cater to the elite of the Upper East Side, offering rejuvenation and relaxation amidst opulent surroundings.

➤ **Curated Flavor Profiles:** Discover the unique flavor combinations that Upper East Siders favor, from antioxidant-rich acai blends to indulgent dark chocolate and hazelnut smoothies. Explore how pairing flavors and textures can turn your daily smoothie into a refined culinary experience.

In the heart of Manhattan's Upper East Side, where Central Park's beauty meets Museum Mile's cultural riches, every sip of a smoothie is an opportunity to embrace the art of living well. Whether you're strolling along the historic streets or sipping in one of the neighborhood's chic cafes, the art of sipping is a cherished tradition among the city's elite. Welcome to The Manhattan Diaries, where savoring a smoothie is as sophisticated as the city itself.

Completed Tasks: Sipping Smoothies Activities

Inspirational Quote

THE SINGLE MOST IMPORTANT THING IN A CHILD'S PERFORMANCE IS THE QUALITY OF THE TEACHER. MAKING SURE A CHILD SPENDS THE MAXIMUM AMOUNT OF TIME WITH INSPIRATIONAL TEACHERS IS THE MOST IMPORTANT THING. — Michael Gove

Action Items: Intentions and Thoughts

Action Items: Intentions and Thoughts

10

Chelsea's Culinary Charms:
Dining Out with Flair, Minus the Caloric Despair

Manhattan, a city where every brick whispers tales of grandeur, and each alley echoes with gourmet secrets. Here, in the heart of the Big Apple, where desires become dreams and dreams take flight, food isn't just sustenance— it's a symphony. Yet, in the city where temptation lurks at every corner, how does one savor without overindulging? How does one dance the night away, knowing their plate carries not just flavor, but flair without the fare?

Imagine: You're meandering through the chic streets of Chelsea, and while the world is captivated by your ensemble, you're lost in thoughts of the divine dinner that awaits. That, my dear, is the Chelsea Culinary Catwalk, a dance between indulgence and insight, where every dish promises decadence without the dread of overdoing.

In this gourmet chapter of The Manhattan Diaries, we journey through Chelsea's best-kept secrets. From the light-as-air appetizers that tantalize without the toll to the main courses that offer a mélange of taste without the weight. Your taste buds will waltz, tango, and salsa, but your silhouette? Forever statuesque.

But remember, this narrative isn't solely about the dishes—it's about the entire dining experience. It's the candle-lit corners, the allure of the ambiance, the stories shared over shared plates. It's about balancing the art of gastronomy with the heart of the city, about dining with depth, desire, and a touch of discernment.

So, accompany me, as we navigate Chelsea's cobbled streets, unearthing eateries that promise a treat without the cheat. Because in Chelsea, dining out isn't just about the food—it's about the story, the statement, the sophistication. Ready your senses for a culinary escapade where every bite is a promise and every meal, a memoir. Welcome to The Manhattan Diaries—

where your plate mirrors the elegance of your persona, and your culinary choices become as iconic as the Chelsea skyline.

Eating Smart in Chelsea

In the heart of Manhattan's bustling Chelsea, where every street corner beckons with culinary temptations, finding the perfect balance between indulgence and restraint is an art. Picture this: You're strolling down the chic streets of Chelsea, and all eyes are on you, not just because of your impeccable style, but because of the savvy way you navigate the culinary landscape. Welcome to the Chelsea Culinary Catwalk, where every bite is a symphony of flavor without the calorie despair. In this exquisite chapter of The Manhattan Diaries, we'll unravel the secrets to dining smart in Chelsea.

➢ **Appetizer Alchemy**: Start your culinary journey with guilt-free appetizers that tantalize your taste buds without compromising your waistline. Chelsea's restaurants offer an array of appetizers that are light on calories but heavy on flavor, ensuring you savor the moment without the guilt.

➢ **Main Course Mastery**: Explore the art of balancing indulgence and health with Chelsea's main course offerings. From vibrant salads to lean protein options, these dishes promise both taste and well-being, allowing you to enjoy your meal without compromising your health goals.

➢ **Dining with Distinction**: It's not just about the food; it's about the entire dining experience. Discover the candle-lit corners, the allure of the ambiance, and the stories shared over shared plates. Chelsea's restaurants provide the perfect backdrop for an evening of culinary delight and sophistication.

➢ **Chelsea's Culinary Charms**: Navigate the cobbled streets of Chelsea and discover eateries that promise decadence without excess. Whether you're in the mood for international cuisine or local delights, Chelsea offers a diverse culinary landscape that caters to every palate.

➤ **Sweet Sensations**: Indulge your sweet tooth with guilt-free dessert options in Chelsea. From fruit-infused delights to inventive low-calorie confections, these desserts offer a satisfying conclusion to your meal without the caloric regret.

➤ **Cocktails with a Twist**: Chelsea's bars and lounges serve up innovative cocktails that are as delightful as they are mindful of your health. Sip on creative libations crafted with fresh ingredients and lower sugar content, allowing you to enjoy your drink without compromising on taste or wellness.

➤ **Farm-to-Table Freshness**: Chelsea's commitment to fresh, locally-sourced ingredients ensures that you enjoy the finest quality produce while supporting local farmers. Explore restaurants that prioritize sustainability and flavor, offering a farm-to-table dining experience that's both responsible and delicious.

➤ **Artistic Ambiance**: Beyond the menu, Chelsea's dining establishments take pride in their artistic and stylish ambiance. From chic decor to thoughtfully designed interiors, these venues provide an immersive dining experience that celebrates the fusion of culinary art and aesthetic beauty.

As you embark on your culinary journey through Chelsea, savor each moment, knowing that you can dine smart without sacrificing style or taste. These carefully curated options ensure that every bite and sip is a testament to your discerning palate and appreciation for the finer things in life. Welcome to The Manhattan Diaries, where dining in Chelsea becomes an exquisite affair of elegance and epicurean delights.

EAT LIKE AN A-LISTER

Completed Tasks: Eating Smart Activities

_____

_____

_____

_____

_____

_____

_____

_____

_____

_____

_____

_____

_____

_____

_____

_____

_____

_____

_____

_____

_____

_____

_____

_____

_____

_____

Inspirational Quote

MASTERCHEF'S IS ABOUT REAL PEOPLE. IT'S ASPIRATIONAL AND INSPIRATIONAL. THERE'S NOTHING SNOBBISH ABOUT IT. — John Torode

Action Items: Intentions and Thoughts

Artful Dining in Chelsea Galleries

Amidst the vibrant tapestry of Manhattan's Chelsea neighborhood, where the worlds of art, culture, and culinary excellence converge, a unique dining experience awaits those who appreciate the finer things in life. In the heart of the art district, galleries aren't the only places showcasing creativity; restaurants here are culinary canvases, and dishes are masterpieces waiting to be savored. Join me on this artistic gastronomic journey through Chelsea, Where every bite is a stroke of genius, and every meal, a masterpiece.

➢ **Palette to Palate**: Chelsea's art-inspired restaurants take the concept of fusion to the next level. Discover eateries that infuse artistic flair into every dish, creating a visual and gastronomic symphony that delights the senses.

➢ **Culinary Expressions**: Explore restaurants where chefs are the true artists, interpreting flavors as their medium. These dining establishments offer innovative, ever-evolving menus that push the boundaries of taste and presentation.

➢ **Gallery Galore**: Dining in Chelsea often means dining amidst art. Visit restaurants that double as art galleries, where you can enjoy exquisite cuisine while surrounded by captivating works of art.

➢ **Theatrical Dining**: In Chelsea, dining is not just about food; it's about the experience. Uncover restaurants that blend gastronomy with theater, offering immersive dining experiences that transport you to a world of culinary enchantment.

➢ **Culinary Performance**: Chelsea's restaurants often blur the lines between dining and performance art. Experience live cooking demonstrations and interactive dining events that elevate your meal to a theatrical spectacle.

➤ **Artisanal Excellence**: Delve into the world of artisanal food and beverages in Chelsea. From handcrafted cocktails to locally sourced, small-batch ingredients, these establishments celebrate the art of craftsmanship in every bite and sip.

➤ **Gallery-Hopping Gastronomy**: Chelsea is renowned for its art galleries, and some restaurants offer curated dining experiences that include guided gallery tours. Immerse yourself in art both on the plate and on the walls as you explore the neighborhood's spirit.

➤ **Seasonal Sensations**: Chelsea's culinary scene embraces the seasons, with menus that change to reflect the freshest ingredients. Discover restaurants that celebrate the bounties of each season, offering a constantly evolving culinary journey that mirrors the changing art exhibitions nearby.

➤ **Sculptural Sweets**: Discover Chelsea's inventive dessert offerings, where pastry chefs craft confections that resemble miniature sculptures. From delicate sugar work to intricately layered pastries, these artistic desserts are almost too beautiful to eat—almost.

➤ **Avant-Garde Ambiance**: Experience dining spaces in Chelsea that are inspired by the avant-garde, with décor as imaginative as the art on display. Whether it's minimalist design or eclectic furnishings, each restaurant's ambiance offers a unique, immersive setting that complements its creative cuisine.

As you dine in these artistic havens, you'll not only savor delectable dishes but also immerse yourself in the rich cultural tapestry of Chelsea. Just as the neighborhood's galleries and landmarks tell a story, so too do these restaurants, where each meal is a chapter in a gastronomic narrative that celebrates the intersection of art, culture, and cuisine. Welcome to The Manhattan Diaries, where dining in Chelsea becomes a canvas for your own culinary adventures.

Completed Tasks: Artful Dining Activities

Inspirational Quote

THE BEST FORM OF FLATTERY IS TO BE ADMIRED, IMITATED OR
RESPECTED. I'VE ALWAYS FELT PROUD THAT OUR FANS LOOK UP TO US OR
FEEL WE ARE INSPIRATIONAL. — Cheryl James

Action Items: Intentions and Thoughts

EAT LIKE AN A-LISTER

Indulgence with a Side of Wellness

Amidst Manhattan's bustling lifestyle, we dive into the dining experiences that combine indulgence with wellness in this chapter of The Manhattan Diaries. From nourishing yet flavorful restaurants to mindful dining practices, we uncover the secrets of Manhattan's wellness culture. Join us in savoring the city's neighborhoods, where every bite celebrates well-being. Indulgence meets style and substance in the heart of Manhattan.

➢ **Manhattan's Wellness Wave**: Dive into Manhattan's thriving wellness culture, Where indulgence and health-consciousness coexist. Explore eateries that prioritize nourishing your body while satisfying your cravings.

➢ **Guilt-Free Gourmet**: Discover restaurants in the heart of Manhattan that serve guilt-free gourmet cuisine. Indulge in dishes that are as delicious as they are nutritious, offering a balance between flavor and well-being.

➢ **Mindful Dining**: Immerse yourself in the world of mindful dining, where every bite is a deliberate act of self-care. Learn how Manhattanites prioritize their mental and physical health while savoring exquisite meals.

➢ **Spa-Inspired Flavors**: Experience the flavors of Manhattan's wellness-focused restaurants, where dishes are inspired by the world of spas and relaxation. Enjoy meals that rejuvenate your body and soul.

➢ **Holistic Hospitality**: Explore restaurants that embrace holistic hospitality, providing not only exceptional food but also an ambiance that promotes relaxation and overall well-being.

➢ **Yoga and Dining Fusion**: Uncover the unique concept of combining yoga or meditation sessions with dining experiences.

Learn how Manhattan's wellness enthusiasts elevate their connection to mind, body, and food.

➤ **Ethical Eating**: Delve into the ethical dining movement in Manhattan, where restaurants prioritize sustainability, ethical sourcing, and eco-conscious practices, ensuring that every meal contributes positively to the planet.

➤ **Wellness Wanderlust**: Experience a journey of wellness wanderlust as you navigate Manhattan's neighborhoods, discovering hidden gems that cater to your well-being. From downtown to uptown, each bite and sip contributes to a healthier and happier you.

➤ **Botanical Beverages**: Sip on Manhattan's finest botanical-infused drinks, crafted with wellness in mind. From adaptogenic teas to herb-infused cocktails, discover how these thoughtfully prepared beverages enhance both flavor and well-being, offering a refreshing twist on mindful sipping.

➤ **Farm-to-Table Fusion**: Discover Manhattan's farm-to-table gems that bring fresh, locally sourced ingredients to your plate. These eateries champion sustainable practices and seasonal menus, delivering vibrant flavors and nutrient-rich dishes straight from local farms, enhancing both taste and wellness with every bite.

In the city that never sleeps, wellness takes center stage, offering residents and visitors alike the opportunity to indulge in delectable cuisine while nurturing their bodies and souls. Manhattan's wellness wave is more than a trend; it's a lifestyle, and this chapter of The Manhattan Diaries invites you to savor every moment. Explore the culinary landscape where wellness meets indulgence, and embark on a journey of self-care, mindful eating, and holistic dining experiences. From guilt-free gourmet to spa-inspired flavors, Manhattan's restaurants are here to nourish your well-being.

Completed Tasks: Indulgence and Wellness Activities

_____
_____
_____
_____
_____
_____
_____
_____
_____
_____
_____
_____
_____
_____
_____
_____
_____
_____
_____
_____
_____
_____
_____
_____
_____

Inspirational Quote

I WANT TO BE AN INSPIRATIONAL MODEL. I WANT PEOPLE TO LOOK AT ME AND SAY, 'WOW, SHE LOOKS HEALTHY.' — Ireland Baldwin

Action Items: Intentions and Thoughts

Chelsea's Culinary Movers and Shakers

In the vibrant district of Chelsea, where creativity thrives and the avant-garde sets the stage, the culinary scene is no exception. Here, among the galleries and studios, the food landscape is an art form in itself. Picture this: You're strolling down the cobblestone streets, not just a spectator of the gallery openings, but a connoisseur of Chelsea's culinary delights, where innovation and flavor reign supreme. This, darling, is the Chelsea Culinary Revolution, where every dish is a canvas, every bite a masterpiece.

➢ **The Gallery Bites**: In Chelsea, darling, dining is an art form. These bites aren't just appetizers; they're creations worthy of any gallery opening. Picture yourself savoring dishes that are as visually stunning as they are delicious. Chelsea's culinary scene is like a never-ending art exhibition, and every bite is a masterpiece.

➢ **A Culinary Soiree: Chelsea's Dining Parties**: Oh, honey, Chelsea knows how to throw a dining party like no other. It's not just about food; it's an entire experience. Imagine being swept up in the vibrant energy of Chelsea's dining scene, where the mingling of flavors mirrors the eclectic mix of its residents. It's a soirée you won't want to miss.

➢ **Gourmet Galleries: Dining in Artistic Ambiance**: Dining in Chelsea isn't just about the food; it's about the atmosphere. These restaurants are like immersive art installations, where the décor is as artistic as the cuisine. You'll dine surrounded by creativity, and every meal becomes a multi-sensory experience.

➢ **Chelsea's Culinary Innovators**: Meet the culinary visionaries who are turning Chelsea into a gastronomic playground. These chefs are pushing the boundaries of what's possible in the world of food. Dining in Chelsea means experiencing innovation on a plate. Get ready to be wowed.

➤ **Delicate Decadence: Desserts Beyond Imagination**: In Chelsea, dessert isn't just an afterthought; it's a grand finale. Indulge in sweet creations that are as artistic as they are delectable. These desserts are like sculptures on your plate, and each bite is a decadent masterpiece.

➤ **Hidden Gems: Chelsea's Culinary Secrets**: Chelsea is full of hidden culinary gems waiting to be discovered. These secret spots offer a taste of the neighborhood's soul, and they're cherished by locals in the know. Prepare for a culinary adventure as you uncover these hidden treasures.

➤ **Dining with the Stars: Celebrity Haunts in Chelsea**: Chelsea isn't just home to art galleries; it's a favorite haunt of celebrities. Rub shoulders with the stars at these exclusive dining spots. Who knows, you might end up dining next to your favorite actor or musician.

➤ **Chelsea's Farm-to-Table Revolution**: Experience the farm-to-table movement in the heart of Manhattan. Chelsea's restaurants are embracing locally sourced, fresh ingredients, and they're redefining what it means to dine sustainably. Enjoy a meal that's not only delicious but also good for the planet.

➤ **Sips of Artistry: Chelsea's Craft Cocktail Scene**: Raise a glass to Chelsea's vibrant cocktail culture, where mixologists blend flavors with the same creativity that fills the art galleries.

As we navigate the culinary world of Chelsea, we'll unravel the stories behind these innovative dishes, the ambiance that complements the creativity, and the culinary pioneers who are shaping the district's dining culture. So, come with me as we dine in the artistic embrace of Chelsea, where every meal is a work of art, and every restaurant a masterpiece in itself. Welcome to The Manhattan Diaries-where the culinary scene is as avant-garde as the galleries that surround it.

Completed Tasks: Movers and Shakers Activities

Action Items: Intentions and Thoughts

Action Items: Intentions and Thoughts

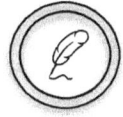

City Roundup: Final Course— A Taste of Manhattan's Soul

As we conclude our captivating journey through the pages of "City Roundup: Final Course—A Taste of Manhattan's Soul," we find ourselves at the intersection of gastronomy and self-discovery, having traversed the enchanting streets of Manhattan in pursuit of both culinary and personal enlightenment.

Throughout the ten vibrant chapters of this book, we've embarked on an epicurean adventure that transcends mere dining; it's a reflection of our deepest desires, a celebration of our aspirations, and a journey into the very core of our existence.

From the chic cobblestone lanes of SoHo to the Upper East Side's elite elixirs, we've indulged our senses in the city's diverse tapestry of flavors, savoring each bite and sip as a testament to life's grandeur. The captivating dance between Manhattan's iconic landmarks and its culinary treasures has revealed that every meal is a statement, every sip an experience, and every bite an affirmation of our connection to this dynamic metropolis.

As you close the final chapter of this book, let it serve as a reminder that the art of dining extends beyond the confines of the plate; it's a celebration of the soul. May your culinary adventures continue to unfold, each bite leading you closer to your inner self, and may the allure of Manhattan and the mysteries within you forever intertwine, creating a symphony of flavors and self-discovery that resonates through every corner of your being. Here's to the enduring enchantment of the city that never sleeps and the unending quest for both culinary and personal fulfillment. Cheers!

Eat Like An A-Lister Recap Checklist

The Manhattan Diaries program series recap checklist—completes step six of your 21 step journey. Think of this program as a time release supplement that does its magic over the course of 21 steps, days, or weeks—you set your schedule. By committing to one chapter each morning—or one book each day or week; in 21 short days or weeks you will be able to change your life into a new You. In this book, we covered:

1. Uptown Greens: Decoding the Salads of the Elite

In this chapter of The Manhattan Diaries, "Uptown Greens," we dive into the chic world of Manhattan's salad culture, where each leaf is carefully curated, and every vinaigrette is a statement. From the timeless Caesar to the trendy frisée, these salads are more than just meals—they're reflections of taste, elegance, and culinary finesse. As we explore the art of upscale dining, we uncover the secrets behind the city's most sophisticated salads and the haute spots where these leafy creations shine. Join us as we revel in the flavors and finesse of uptown eating, discovering how every bite in Manhattan becomes an exquisite expression of style and discernment.

2. Madison Avenue Munchies: Snacking with Style and Substance

In this chapter of The Manhattan Diaries, "Madison Avenue Munchies," we explore the sophisticated art of snacking with style in the heart of Manhattan. As we stroll along Madison Avenue, where every nibble becomes a statement, we delve into the city's chicest treats—from delicate, melt-in-your-mouth macarons to bold, savory bites that embody flair and finesse. Here, snacking isn't merely about indulgence; it's about capturing the city's essence through flavors, textures, and carefully chosen treats that reveal a story of taste, ambition, and elegance. Join us on this culinary journey, where every bite is an ode to Manhattan's unique charm and allure.

3. Central Park Picnics: Alfresco Dining with a Gourmet Twist

In this chapter of The Manhattan Diaries, "Central Park Picnic Panache," we dive into the art of crafting a posh, unforgettable picnic in the heart of Manhattan. Set against the iconic skyline, this is no ordinary meal; it's a performance of elegance and epicurean delight. From delicately marinated olives to artisanal cheeses and bubbly, every detail of your spread is designed to captivate and charm. As you embrace the harmony of Central Park's natural beauty with Manhattan's upscale flair, you create a dining experience that's as stylish and spontaneous as the city itself. This is alfresco dining at its finest—an invitation to savor sophistication under the open sky.

4. Broadway Bites: Power Breakfasts to Kickstart Your Day

In The Manhattan Diaries chapter "Broadway Bites: Power Breakfasts to Kickstart Your Day," we explore the energizing breakfasts that fuel Manhattan's ambitious spirit. Here, mornings are more than a meal; they're a stage for setting the day's tempo with style and vigor. From vibrant smoothies to creative avocado toasts, each bite prepares you for the city's daily theater of dreams and determination. With sustenance as sophisticated as a Broadway debut, breakfast becomes a ritual of ambition and elegance, readying you to step into the rhythm of the bustling city.

5. Fifth Avenue Feasts: Dinners Worthy of the Front Row at Fashion Week

In The Manhattan Diaries chapter "Fifth Avenue Feasts: Dinners Worthy of the Front Row at Fashion Week," dining in Manhattan becomes an art form, blending opulence with elegance in the city's most elite establishments. This chapter takes you on a journey through Manhattan's grand dining experiences on Fifth Avenue, where each dish is as exquisite as haute couture. From truffles and champagne to ambiance and conversation, every detail embodies sophistication. Here, dinner isn't just about the meal; it's a sensory symphony that mirrors the city's flair for style and luxury, leaving an indelible mark on the Manhattan dining scene.

6. SoHo Sips: Luxurious Liquids and Decadent Drinks for the Discerning Palate

In the chapter "SoHo Sips: Luxurious Liquids and Decadent Drinks for the Discerning Palate" of The Manhattan Diaries, we journey into the heart of Manhattan's most stylish and sophisticated drink culture. Here, in SoHo's iconic bars and intimate speakeasies, each sip is an experience—blending vintage wines that evoke the past with cocktails that sparkle with the future. More than taste, these drinks embody the city's spirit, where every clink of a glass tells a story, invites company, and radiates the charm of Manhattan's most chic hideaways. It's a celebration of indulgence, where each glass captures the city's elegance and creativity.

7. Manhattan's Midnight Indulgences: Guilt-Free Treats for After Hours

In the chapter "Manhattan's Midnight Indulgences: Guilt-Free Treats for After Hours" of The Manhattan Diaries, we explore Manhattan's enchanting world of late-night delights, where each treat offers a taste of indulgence without the guilt. Strolling through the moonlit streets of the West Village, from creamy vegan chocolates to airy macarons, these after-dark bites are crafted with elegance and allure. It's about the ambiance as much as the flavor, an experience that captures the city's nighttime magic and nourishes the soul. In Manhattan, every midnight snack becomes a memorable part of the city's late-night allure.

8. West Village Wellness: Superfoods to Keep You Glowing from Within

In "West Village Wellness: Superfoods to Keep You Glowing from Within," The Manhattan Diaries takes readers on a journey through the West Village, Manhattan's haven for health and vitality. Here, amidst its cobblestone charm and holistic cafés, wellness is a lifestyle, from antioxidant-rich matcha lattes to nutrient-packed chia puddings. It's more than just nourishment; it's a celebration of inner radiance that shines through in every smile and step. In this tranquil corner of the city, wellness becomes an art form, offering a glow that's rooted as much in the heart as it is in Manhattan's vibrant rhythm.

9. East Side Elixirs: Smoothies and Juices the Celebs Won't Stop Talking About

In "East Side Elixirs: Smoothies and Juices the Celebs Won't Stop Talking About," The Manhattan Diaries unveils the world of the Upper East Side's trendiest health elixirs, where smoothies and juices are as stylish as they are nourishing. From luxurious avocado blends for flawless skin to vibrant berry concoctions adored by A-listers, these drinks embody the elegance and wellness balance Manhattan's elite crave. More than just nutrition, each sip is a statement of opulence, a taste of the exclusive East Side lifestyle. In this chapter, the city's most glamorous greens and revitalizing reds reveal the secrets behind their radiant allure.

10. Chelsea's Culinary Charms: Dining Out with Flair, Minus the Calorie Despair

In "Chelsea's Culinary Charms: Dining Out with Flair, Minus the Caloric Despair," The Manhattan Diaries guides readers through Chelsea's chic dining scene, where indulgence meets balance. This chapter reveals the secrets of Chelsea's refined eateries, where each dish offers sophistication without the burden of excess. From airy appetizers to artful main courses, the dining experience here is a graceful dance of taste and mindfulness. Amidst candle-lit ambiance and shared stories, readers will discover how Chelsea brings flavor, elegance, and restraint together, allowing them to savor every bite in true Manhattan style.

Where Do We Go From Here?

Darlings, as we conclude our glamorous journey through the world of "Eat Like an A-Lister: Manhattan's Ultimate Nutrition Guide," we find ourselves standing at a crossroads in this dazzling city, wondering, "Where Do We Go from Here?"

Throughout these pages, we've unveiled the secrets to creating an allure that's as iconic as the Manhattan skyline itself. From the twinkling dewy dawn look to the sultry nighttime shimmer, we've embraced every facet of Manhattan's mystique. We've learned that makeup is not just a mask; it's an expression, a statement of our inner selves.

But the magic doesn't end with the final page of this book. No, my dears, it's merely the beginning. Manhattan is a city of reinvention, where change is not only embraced but celebrated. As we navigate the intricate streets and charming neighborhoods, let's carry the lessons of this journey with us.

Where do we go from here? We go forward with confidence, grace, and the knowledge that the beauty we seek is already within us. Manhattan may dazzle with its lights, but it's you who shines the brightest. Whether you're strolling through Central Park, closing deals on Wall Street, or sipping cocktails at a rooftop bar, let your inner allure radiate.

So, embrace the city's ever-changing pulse, seize the opportunities that lie ahead, and continue writing your own Manhattan diaries. Remember, it's not about where you've been; it's about where you're headed. And in the city that never sleeps, the possibilities are as limitless as your dreams.

As we part ways, take a piece of Manhattan's mystique with you, for it's an everlasting part of your story. Keep mesmerizing the world with your inner self, your style, and your indomitable spirit. The Manhattan allure never fades; it merely evolves. Embrace that evolution, embrace yourself, and let the city's mystique guide you to new heights.

Until we meet again under the shimmering lights of Manhattan, my darlings, remember that the journey is just as enchanting as the destination. So, go forth and continue to mesmerize the world, one captivating chapter at a time.

EAT LIKE AN A-LISTER

Completed Tasks: Recap Checklist Activities

_____

_____
_____
_____
_____
_____
_____
_____
_____
_____
_____
_____
_____
_____
_____
_____
_____
_____
_____
_____
_____
_____
_____
_____
_____
_____

Inspirational Quote

ONLY I CAN CHANGE MY LIFE. NO ONE CAN DO IT FOR ME. — Carol Burnett

CITY ROUNDUP

Action Items: Intentions and Thoughts

Journal Pages: Pen Your Tales

COCKTAILS & CHRONICLES

Journal Pages: Pen Your Tales

Journal Pages: Pen Your Tales

Journal Pages: Pen Your Tales

Journal Pages: Pen Your Tales

Journal Pages: Pen Your Tales

Journal Pages: Pen Your Tales

Journal Pages: Pen Your Tales

Journal Pages: Pen Your Tales

www.ingramcontent.com/pod-product-compliance
Lightning Source LLC
Chambersburg PA
CBHW032054020426
42335CB00011B/328